Health Risks

Elliott J. Howard, M.D.
Internist/Cardiologist at Lenox Hospital
with Susan A. Roth, B.S., M.S.

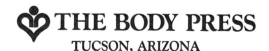

THE BODY PRESS
TUCSON, ARIZONA

Dedication

I dedicate this book to my father, Robert L. Howard (1894-1978), whose life as Director and Founder of Camp Seneca for boys and girls was dedicated to the dictum of Aurelius Seneca, "mens sana in corpore sano—a sound mind in a sound body."

Published by The Body Press
A Division of HPBooks, Inc.
P.O. Box 5367
Tucson, AZ 85703
(602) 888-2150

ISBN: 0-89586-442-8 (hardback)
ISBN: 0-89586-484-3 (paperback)
Library of Congress Catalog Card Number: 86-70418
© 1986 Elliott J. Howard, M.D., and Susan A. Roth
Printed in U.S.A.
1st Printing

CONTENTS

About the Authors

For 25 years, Elliott J. Howard, M.D., F.A.C.P., F.A.C.C., has belonged to the medical staff of Lenox Hill Hospital and has practiced internal medicine and cardiology in New York City. His interest in preventive medicine began early in his career, when he taught medicine and was a research fellow investigating cholesterol metabolism and atherosclerosis at Columbia University College of Physicians and Surgeons.

In 1970, Dr. Howard established the Foundation for Study of Exercise, Stress and the Heart to investigate Americans' health habits as they relate to development of heart disease. His clinical research has been published in the *American Heart Journal, Circulation, Journal of the American Medical Association, Diseases of the Chest, Angiology* and other medical journals.

Dr. Howard is a fellow of the American College of Physicians, the American College of Cardiology and the American College of Sports Medicine. He is on the board of directors of the New York County Medical Society and chairman of its Committee on Continuing Education. Dr. Howard is also a member of the board of governors of New York's City Athletic Club, consulting cardiologist for the New York State Disability Services and associate medical director of the Cardiometric Institute, as well as being the medical director of the Foundation for Study of Exercise, Stress and the Heart. Formerly Dr. Howard was attending physician at the Bronx Veterans Administration Hospital, attending cardiologist at St. Barnabas Hospital and a member of the American Federation for Clinical Research.

Dr. Howard has long believed that good nutrition, vigorous exercise and stress reduction play major roles in disease prevention. He practices what he believes and participates actively in squash, tennis, downhill skiing and cross-country skiing.

Susan A. Roth has been an editor with a New York publishing house and a magazine editor. She now works as a freelance writer, specializing in health and gardening. She holds a bachelor's degree and a master's degree from Cornell University.

Ms. Roth recently completed a health book about arthritis, and her writing has appeared in national magazines. She has also written for Rodale Press, Ortho Books and World Book. Also a professional photographer, Ms. Roth's garden photography has appeared in calendars and gardening books.

A believer in good nutrition and preventive health, Ms. Roth walks regularly, takes aerobics classes and enjoys hiking, canoeing, cross-country skiing and gardening.

INTRODUCTION

In the early years of my medical practice, it became evident to me that many people were eating themselves into premature death. I began working on a semihumorous diet book titled "Food Kills." I had been a Research Fellow at Columbia University College of Physicians and Surgeons, working with a group of physicians (Doctors David Seegal, Arthur Wertheim, Quentin Deming, Alfred Steiner, Forrest Kendall, Liese Abell and Dan Rudman) studying cholesterol and its relationship to atherosclerosis. I was convinced cholesterol and fat in the diet contributed to development of heart disease. This was in the 1960s when carbohydrate was a "dirty word," protein was all good and could do no harm, and fat wasn't so bad (a la Atkins, Tarnower and others).

As research and better understanding of good nutrition developed, it became evident the opposite was true—the most nutritious foods were carbohydrates (vegetables and fruits taken in variety). And while protein was important, it should be eaten in the lowest-fat form, in a fraction of the quantity we had grown accustomed to. And we discovered cholesterol really was important.

My focus then turned to describing a nutritious diet, but because obesity and overweight were rampant (and so were diet books), I focused on the psychological aspect of analyzing why people overate and advising them how to control the stress that drove them to it. I collaborated with N.Y.U. Psychiatry Professor George Serban, M.D., and began work on a diet-stress advice book. Meanwhile, diet books were springing up like weeds—many worthless and unhealthy but some sound and worthwhile. Therefore, I became interested in analyzing all the important risk factors that can harm one's health.

The research of my Foundation for Study of Exercise, Stress and the Heart was a useful starting point. Collation of pertinent data from many large national and international epidemiology studies with work I had already done has resulted in this book.

I am convinced poor eating habits is a major cause of ill health; finding the right balance, eliminating certain foods and emphasizing others can be an important preventive measure, especially against heart disease and cancer! I am further convinced exercise is a benefit in many aspects of our lives; stress combined with other bad habits is a major influence in development of heart disease.

Special thanks go to Peter Ryan, Jon Latimer and Dr. Wilbur James Gould for their advice and encouragement, which led to the idea for this book. Others I am indebted to for major support in my studies include Simon and Kitty Aldewereld, Alan Fortunoff, Marie-Louise Garbaty, Charles Greenebaum, Fay Imerblum, Jacques Leviant, Mark Millard, M. Hughes Miller, Robert Raisler, Anthony Ritter, Robert Wetenhall, Gene Woodfin and Paul Woolard. Thanks to Judith Knorr for analyzing the menus for the risk-reducing nutrition plan. Special acknowledgment for advice, research and editing goes to Susan A. Roth.

The writing and research for this book were supported by the Foundation for Study of Exercise, Stress and the Heart. I wish to thank Lorraine Rubenstein for secretarial help and Annette Avitabile for technical assistance.

Elliott J. Howard, M.D., F.A.C.P., F.A.C.C.
New York City
July 7, 1986

PART I.

EVALUATE YOUR RISKS

1.
YOUR HIDDEN HEALTH RISKS

Most of us feel lucky to live in one of the richest countries in the world. We have immense personal freedom, our housing is luxurious, our diet is extravagant, our jobs are fulfilling and not physically strenuous, and our health care is superior. That should mean we live longer, healthier lives than less-fortunate people. Right? Wrong!

It is because of all these "luxuries" that we have the second-highest heart-attack rate in the world and our cancer rates are high! If you're not concerned about suddenly finding yourself with a serious heart disease or cancer, wake up! If you're an average person leading an ordinary life, odds are fairly high you'll develop heart disease or cancer long before you're "ready to go." You may be able to do something *now* to protect yourself and maybe even prevent the disease.

From 1850 to 1950, the life expectancy of North Americans *doubled,* largely because of improved sanitation, a decrease in infant mortality and the development of antibiotics to control infectious diseases. When infectious diseases no longer threatened our lives, cancer, heart disease and stroke were left to kill us off. Despite advances we have made in medical understanding and treatment of these diseases since 1950, there has been no significant improvement in our life expectancy.

A major 5-year study, conducted by the Carter Center at Emory University, revealed the 14 primary causes of illness and premature death (death before age 65). The six risk factors most frequently cited were *tobacco, alcohol, injuries, unintended pregnancy, lack of preventive service* and *poor nutrition.* Tobacco was identified as the single leading cause of death—1,000 deaths *each day* are attributed to tobacco!

Alcohol was the second most important risk factor, and poor nutrition was also a leading risk factor.

You don't have to be on the wrong side of statistics! You have the opportunity to take control over many of these risk factors of premature death. Alcohol, tobacco and poor nutrition don't have to kill you. You can take steps now to help you live a long, vigorous life, staying healthy and active well into your 80s and even 90s.

WHAT IS KILLING US?

The two most common illnesses that kill us are *arteriosclerosis* (commonly called *hardening of the arteries)* and *cancer.* Arteriosclerosis of the heart, kidneys and brain causes heart attack, hypertension (high blood pressure) and stroke. Cancers of the lung, colon, breast, pancreas and prostate are the most frequent killer cancers. See illustration below.

The seven countries with the highest rates of breast cancer (over 20 breast-cancer deaths per 100,000 deaths a year) are the same countries where people eat the highest amounts of fat—150 grams (about 1/3 pound) or more a day. People who live in the seven countries with the lowest rates of breast cancer (less than 5 per 100,000 a year) eat the lowest amounts of dietary fat—less than 50 grams a day.

The story for heart disease is similar. Wealthier countries with higher standards of living and "tastier" diets lead all other countries in deaths from heart attacks. Last year, 1.5 million people in the United States suffered heart attacks—another 500,000 died from heart disease. Every day, 1,200 Americans die from a sudden, unexpected heart attack. Cardiovascular disease is the *leading* cause of death in the industrialized Western world.

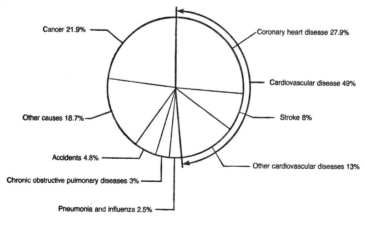

Present causes of death among Americans. Based on data from the National Center for Health Statistics.

3

Scientific studies show when people from low-risk countries immigrate to the United States, protection from these diseases is short-lived. As these people become "Americanized" and adopt a new diet and lifestyle, they become susceptible to the same diseases that kill us.

YOU DON'T HAVE TO BE A STATISTIC

If you're like the rest of us, you want to live a long, happy, healthy life and die only when you're "ready to go." But what are you doing now to help ensure you don't drop dead tomorrow? If you're like most people, you live as if there is nothing you can do to help yourself. You hope fate will treat you fairly. You act as if your destiny is out of your hands.

When a sudden, massive heart attack strikes a friend or co-worker, or someone you know suffers a slow death from cancer, you shake your head and say, "What bad luck!" But you shudder inwardly to think fate may hand you the same raw deal, and you wish fervently that scientists could develop a cure for cancer and heart disease before you need it.

Living in our industrialized world doesn't predestine you to cancer or heart disease. It's *you,* not luck, that has the greatest control over your health. Science has shown each person has an individual, measurable risk of being stricken by disease; some of your risk is within your control! That means you can control your "health destiny." Learn which risk factors affect your health and decrease your odds of dying young from a critical disease, then change your habits to minimize those risk factors.

Your goal should be to prevent damage by disease and to protect your essential body organs so they'll endure in top functioning condition. You can't abuse your vital organs and realistically expect to avoid disease.

The problem of prevention is largely up to you, and few of us want to make the sacrifices involved or admit we are vulnerable. But why risk your breasts or your heart for a cheese Danish? Why risk your lungs and your life for a cigarette? The sacrifices aren't really so great when you consider the alternatives!

I ask my patients, "Why wait until you need a cure when prevention is easier and more desirable? Would you rather suffer the miserable side effects of chemotherapy, lose parts of your body to a surgeon, wear a colostomy bag for the rest of your life or change your lifestyle now?" Which would you choose?

YOU'RE GAMBLING WITH YOUR LIFE

Many people approach their health with what I like to call the "quick-buck" approach. They seek and expect a quick miracle cure for whatever ails them and often gamble with their health. I'm dismayed by the popularity and best-seller status of books that promote wild, unconventional—and medically dangerous—diets, fitness

4

programs and disease cures. These books, which promise a few quick, easy steps to lose weight, stop aging, cure arthritis, cure cancer or prevent heart disease, help no one except the publishers and the authors.

Would you gamble with your life? Anyone who continually follows the latest health fad promoted by a pseudoscientist (whose recommendations are not based on sound scientific studies) is gambling with his life and his health. You shouldn't ingest large quantities of any substances—vitamins, minerals or herbs—because some authority promises it's an easy, painless way to lose weight or extend your life.

Play it safe—be wary of any miracle cures. Listen to the findings and advice that come from scientifically proven studies, even if they promise no miracles or quick cures. In the long run, you won't be seeking the next quick cure because you won't need one. Scientific research has advanced our knowledge of the human body to such an extent that it's possible for almost anyone to alter the course of his life and lower risks of cancer, heart disease, stroke and other diseases.

If you decide to follow a quick-fix regime rather than listen to what scientists and medical professionals are saying, then you may pay the price. If you decide to wait until all the proof is in, it may be too late to take advantage of what scientists already know.

The following research findings, which I discuss in more detail in later sections, are facts we now know about leading diseases that cause death in the United States.

- Men who have physically active jobs have less coronary-artery disease than men with sedentary jobs.
- People who smoke 1-1/2 packs of cigarettes a day have twice the rate of fatal heart attacks as non-smokers.
- Certain laboratory animals, bred to be highly susceptible to cancer, get less cancer than expected when exercised and kept lean on a high-carbohydrate diet.
- Sudden cardiac arrest occurs 4 times more frequently in obese people (those 30% or more above their ideal weight) than it does in people closer to ideal weight.
- Lowering the average serum-cholesterol level in an experimental group by 10% lowers the group's incidence of coronary disease by 23%.
- Brain scans of people who drink alcohol heavily on a daily basis show their brains slowly atrophy.
- Drinking more than 3 ounces of hard liquor a day is associated with an increased death rate from cancer. Drinkers who smoke have the highest rates.
- Men who are 20% overweight live 20% shorter lives than normal-weight men. Women who are 20% overweight live 10% shorter lives than normal-weight women.
- Fat consumption has been directly linked to the rate of colon cancer, the second most common form of cancer in the United States.
- A study of thousands of healthy men, aged 40 to 49, who had normal blood pressure, but who had high cholesterol or smoked, showed those who stopped

smoking and lowered their cholesterol by improving their diet had 47% fewer heart attacks and deaths from sudden cardiac arrest.

● Advances in medical research on atherosclerosis during the past 10 years have helped decrease the death rate from heart disease by 25% and the death rate from stroke by 40%.

These findings offer some clues about how risk factors determine your chances of developing a major illness. Even with the medical discoveries scientists have made, it's still up to you to keep yourself from falling on the wrong side of the statistics!

YOU CAN CHANGE YOUR RISK FACTORS

Take the risk-factor longevity test that begins on the following page to see how much your present lifestyle may be affecting your health and shortening your life. Then read the sections that discuss the particular risk factors of heart disease, cancers and other problems.

Included in this book are specific risk-factor tests that you can take to help you determine the odds of suffering a particular illness, such as diabetes, osteoporosis, colon cancer, lung cancer, stroke and other diseases. Take the tests, then consider the results. If you're not at risk, you're doing something right. If you are at risk, it's never too late to change.

I want to teach you to help lower your risks of cancer, heart disease and other life-threatening illnesses. I provide you with a risk-reducing nutrition plan that may lower your risks. See page 186. If you're overweight, you can learn how to lose weight permanently, without risk; see page 204. And I provide you with a risk-reducing exercise plan that may add years to your life. See page 226.

If you follow the advice I give my patients, many of them prominent New York professionals and show-business personalities, you'll know you're doing something to protect your health and vigor. You can rest assured you're helping yourself live a life relatively free from the major diseases that strike us.

You may be able to do more than just *beat the odds*—you may live a longer, healthier, more rewarding life free of cancer, heart disease and other serious illnesses.

TAKE THIS TEST TO MEASURE YOUR LONGEVITY

Your lifestyle choices play a significant role in your overall health and longevity. They are often the key factors in determining whether you develop heart disease, cancer, diabetes, osteoporosis or some other life-threatening condition. If you answer this test honestly, and if you have no obvious symptoms of heart disease, cancer or diabetes, your answers will give you a fairly good evaluation of your expected longevity. If you don't like what the test predicts about your health, this book will tell you how you can take charge and help lower your risks.

Circle the score for each characteristic that applies to you. Total the score, then check your risk category on page 12.

Family History

Choose any that apply.

- −2 Both mother and father were free of cancer and heart disease and lived beyond age 75
- −1 Only one parent was free of cancer and heart disease and lived beyond age 75
- +2 Coronary heart disease before age 50 in one or both parents
- +3 Coronary heart disease before age 40 in one or both parents
- +2 High blood pressure before age 50 in only one parent
- +3 High blood pressure before age 50 in both parents
- +1 Diabetes mellitus before age 60 in one or both parents
- +2 Cancer in a parent or sibling
- +2 Stroke before age 60 in only one parent
- +3 Stroke before age 60 in both parents

Weight

Choose one.

- 0 Normal or within 10% of normal
- +2 Overweight by 20 to 29%
- +3 Overweight by 30 to 39%
- +4 More than 40% overweight

Blood Pressure

Systolic

Choose one.
- −1   100 to 120
- 0   121 to 140
- +1   141 to 170
- +2   171 to 190
- +3   Over 190

Diastolic

Choose one.
- −1   60 to 70
- 0   71 to 85
- +1   86 to 100
- +2   101 to 110
- +3   111 to 120
- +4   Over 120

Cholesterol

Total

Choose one.
- −2   150 to 170
- −1   171 to 190
- 0   191 to 210
- +1   211 to 240
- +2   241 to 280
- +3   281 to 320
- +4   Over 320

HDL

Choose one.
- −2   66 to 80
- −1   51 to 65
- 0   41 to 50
- +1   31 to 40
- +2   25 to 30
- +3   Below 25

Smoking

Choose any that apply.
- −1   Never smoked
- −1   Quit over 5 years ago
- 0   Quit 1 to 5 years ago
- +1   Quit within the past year
- +2   Smoke less than 1 pack of cigarettes a day
- +3   Smoke 1 pack of cigarettes a day
- +4   Smoke about 1-1/2 packs of cigarettes a day
- +5   Smoke 2 packs of cigarettes a day
- +1   Smoke a pipe or cigars
- +3   Began smoking as a teenager
- +5   Have smoked for more than 20 years
- +1   Smoke marijuana 1 or 2 times a week
- +2   Smoke marijuana daily
- +1   Live *or* work in heavily air-polluted area
- +2   Live *and* work in heavily air-polluted area

Alcohol Use

Choose any that apply.
- −1 Drink no more than 1-1/2 ounces of hard liquor, 12 ounces of beer or 5 ounces of wine once or twice a week
- 0 Drink almost every day but not more than 1-1/2 ounces of hard liquor, 12 ounces of beer or 5 ounces of wine a day
- +1 Drink two drinks each day totalling 3 ounces of hard liquor, 24 ounces of beer or 10 ounces of wine
- +2 Drink more than two drinks each day
- +5 Smoke cigarettes, pipe or cigar, and drink alcohol at least several times a week

Personality and Stress Evaluation

Choose any that apply.
- +1 Intense desire to get ahead
- +2 Constant driving need for success
- +2 Easily irritated, annoyed or frustrated
- +2 Angry and hostile if losing in competition
- +2 Fiercely competitive; must win
- +3 Angry and hostile, even if successful
- +1 Have many projects going on at once
- +1 Constantly bothered by incomplete work
- +2 Don't express anger; hold feelings inside
- +2 Work hard without feeling satisfaction
- +2 Frequent stress symptoms—knot in stomach, heart palpitations, headaches, poor sleep, intestinal symptoms, constipation
- +2 Hardly laugh; depressed often
- +2 Rarely discuss problems or feelings with others
- +2 Constantly strive to please others rather than yourself
- −1 None of the above

Exercise

Choose one in each group, then calculate your score for this section as indicated on page 10.

Frequency of Exercise
- +5 Daily or almost daily
- +4 3 to 5 times a week
- +3 1 to 2 times a week
- +2 2 to 3 times a month
- +1 Less than 3 times a month

Duration of Each Exercise Period
+4   More than 45 minutes
+3   20 to 40 minutes
+2   10 to 20 minutes
+1   Less than 10 minutes

Intensity of Each Exercise Period
+5   Sustained vigorous exercise
+4   Intermittent vigorous exercise
+3   Moderately vigorous exercise
+2   Moderately non-vigorous exercise
+1   Light, leisurely activity

To determine your fitness rating, multiply your score for each section.

_____ X	_____ X	_____ =	_____
Intensity	Duration	Frequency	Score

For example: 3 x 4 x 3 = 36. The maximum is 100. Use your answer to determine your physical-fitness rating below.

Physical-Fitness Rating

Choose one.
−2   81-100 is very active, high fitness
−1   61-80 is active and healthy
 0   41-60 is acceptable and good
+1   31-40 is not good enough
+2   21-30 is inadequate
+3   20 and below is sedentary, poor fitness

Dietary Habits

Choose any that apply.
+2   Use salt freely, without tasting food first
+2   Eat cabbage, broccoli or cauliflower less than 3 times a week
+3   Eat high-fiber grains, such as whole-wheat bread, brown rice and bran cereal, less than once a day
+3   Eat fewer than 3 fruits and vegetables a day
+1   Follow a fad weight-loss diet once or twice a year

Eat heartily at meals, and snack between meals:
+ 3   Daily or almost daily
+ 2   4 days a week
+ 1   2 days a week

Eat beef, bacon or processed meats:
+ 3   5 to 6 times a week
+ 2   4 times a week
+ 1   2 times a week

Eat eggs, alone or in other foods:
+ 3   12 eggs a week
+ 2   8 eggs a week
+ 1   6 eggs a week

Eat ice cream, cake or rich desserts:
+ 2   Almost every day
+ 1   Several times a week

Eat butter, cream, cream cheese and cheese:
+ 3   Every day
+ 2   Almost every day
+ 1   2 to 3 times a week

Sex and Physical Build

Choose one.
    0   Male, with slim build
+ 1   Male, heavily muscled, with stocky build
+ 3   Female, take birth-control pills and smoke
+ 1   Female, post-menopausal and take estrogen
    0   Female, take birth-control pills and don't smoke
    0   Female, post-menopausal and don't take estrogen

INTERPRETING YOUR SCORE

To determine your score, add all scores from the categories. Check your total score below to see if your health and your life are at risk. You may be referred to the risk-reducing nutrition plan, page 186, or the risk-reducing exercise plan, page 226.

−15   **Lowest Risk**—This is the best possible score. You should enjoy a long, healthy life free of cancer, heart disease, stroke or diabetes.

−14 to +6   **Low Risk**—You are in very good health; odds are in your favor of continued good health and a long, productive life free of cancer, heart disease, diabetes and stroke. If you wish to improve your odds, check the test to see where you gained points. If possible, work on improving those areas.

7 to 11   **Moderate Risk**—You are at some risk of developing ill-health and can expect to live an average life span. Try to correct conditions or habits for which you scored a 2, 3 or 4, and you may help add years to your life. Stop smoking, if you smoke, and follow the risk-reducing nutrition plan and risk-reducing exercise plan. These will help lower your risks.

12 to 20   **High Risk**—Your risk of developing a life-threatening illness early in life and dying sooner than you should is considerable. You can help lower your risks by correcting conditions for which you scored a 2, 3 or 4. Stop smoking, if you smoke, and follow the risk-reducing nutrition plan and the risk-reducing exercise plan to help lower your risks.

21+   **Very High Risk**—Your health is at dangerous risk, and you may die prematurely if you don't change your ways immediately to begin to correct your unhealthy habits. Seek medical advice and psychological therapy to help you change your habits. Stop smoking, if you smoke, and follow the risk-reducing nutrition plan and the risk-reducing exercise plan to help lower your risks.

2.

IS YOUR
HEART AT RISK?

*TAKE THIS TEST TO MEASURE YOUR
HEART-DISEASE RISK*

This test measures your risk of developing heart disease. Tests in the following sections pinpoint additional risk factors about which you may need to be concerned. Circle the score for each characteristic that applies to you. Total the score, then check your risk category on page 17.

Personal

Choose one in each of the following statements.
Your sex and age is:

    0   Woman younger than 55
 +1   Man younger than 55
 +2   Woman 55 or older
 +3   Man 55 to 65
 +4   Man 65 or older

Among your close blood relatives, there have been heart attacks:

    0   In no parent, grandparent, aunt or uncle before age 60
 +1   In one or more parents, grandparents, aunts or uncles
         after age 60

+2   In one parent, grandparent, aunt or uncle before age 60
+3   In two of the above relatives before age 60
+4   In more than two of the above relatives before age 60

Among your close blood relatives, the following medical conditions existed:

  0   No serious high blood pressure, diabetes or high cholesterol
+1   Serious high blood pressure, diabetes or high cholesterol in only one close relative
+2   Serious high blood pressure, diabetes or high cholesterol in two close relatives
+3   Serious high blood pressure, diabetes or high cholesterol in more than two close relatives

Cholesterol

Choose one in each of the following statements.

Your serum-cholesterol level is:

   0   190 or below
 +2   191 to 230
 +6   231 to 289
+12   290 to 319
+16   Over 320

Your HDL-cholesterol is:

 −2   Over 60
  0   45 to 60
 +2   35 to 44
 +6   29 to 34
+12   23 to 28
+16   Below 23

Smoking

Choose one in each of the following statements.
You have smoked now or in the past:

  0   Never smoked, or quit over 5 years ago
+2   Quit 2 to 4 years ago
+3   Quit about 1 year ago
+6   Quit during the past year

The number of cigarettes you now smoke is:

+9   1/2 to 1 pack a day

+12 1 to 2 packs a day
+15 More than 2 packs a day

The quality of the air you breath is:

  0   Unpolluted by smoke, exhaust or industry at home *and* at work
+2 Live *or* work with smokers in unpolluted area
+4 Live *and* work with smokers in unpolluted area
+6 Live *or* work with smokers *and* live or work in air-polluted area
+8 Live *and* work with smokers *and* live and work in air-polluted area

Blood Pressure

Choose one.
Your blood pressure is:

  0   120/75 or below
 +2 120/75 to 140/85
 +6 140/85 to 150/90
 +8 150/90 to 175/100
+10 175/100 to 190/110
+12 190/110 or above

Exercise

Choose one.
Your exercise habits are:

  0   Exercise vigorously 4 or 5 times a week
+2 Exercise moderately 4 or 5 times a week
+4 Exercise only on weekends
+6 Exercise occasionally
+8 Little or no exercise

Weight

Choose one.
Your weight history is:

  0   Always at, or near, ideal weight
+1 Presently 10% overweight
+2 Presently 20% overweight
+3 Presently 30% or more overweight
+4 Presently 20% or more overweight and have been since before age 30

Stress

Choose one.
You feel overstressed:
- 0   Rarely at work or at home
- +3   Somewhat at home but not at work
- +5   Somewhat at work but not at home
- +7   Somewhat at work *and* home
- +9   Almost constantly at work *or* home
- +12   Almost constantly at work *and* home

Diabetes

Choose one.
Your diabetic history is:
- 0   Blood sugar has always been normal
- +2   Slightly elevated blood glucose (prediabetic) or slightly low (hypoglycemic)
- +4   Diabetic beginning after age 40 requiring strict dietary or insulin control
- +5   Diabetic beginning before age 30 requiring strict dietary or insulin control

Alcohol

Choose one.
You drink alcoholic beverages:
- 0   Never, or only socially, about once or twice a month or only one 5-ounce glass of wine or 12-ounce glass of beer or 1-1/2 ounces of hard liquor about 5 times a week
- +2   Two to three 5-ounce glasses of wine or 12-ounce glasses of beer or 1-1/2-ounce cocktails about 5 times a week
- +4   Drink more than three 1-1/2-ounce cocktails or more than three 5-ounce glasses of wine or 12-ounce glasses of beer almost every day

INTERPRETING YOUR SCORE

To determine your score, add all scores from the categories. Check your total score below to see if your health and your life are at risk.

0 to 20	**Low Risk**—Your family history and lifestyle habits are excellent; your risk of heart disease is probably minimal.
21 to 50	**Moderate Risk**—Your family history or lifestyle habits are putting you at moderate risk. You may lower your risks and minimize your genetic predisposition if you change any poor habits.
51 to 74	**High Risk**—Your family history and lifestyle habits are responsible for your high risk of heart disease. Change your habits now to help lower your risk.
75 +	**Very High Risk**—Your family history and a lifetime of poor habits are putting you at very high risk of heart disease. Eliminate as many factors as you can to help lower risks.

Is Your Heart at Risk?

In 1985, nearly 1 million men and women in the United States died from cardiovascular disease, and 1-1/2 million more had non-fatal heart attacks. Every day of the year, 1,200 Americans die from "sudden cardiac arrest." Forty-two million others are affected with some form of cardiovascular disease; only 8 million have obvious symptoms, such as chest pain, shortness of breath or calf pains when walking. The remaining 32 million don't even know they're in danger!

About 2-1/2 times as many men as women are victims of heart disease, although the incidence of heart disease among women has steadily risen during the past decades. Equal numbers of blacks and whites are affected.

As bleak as these numbers may seem, it's even sadder to realize most people represented by these statistics don't really have to be among those stricken—at least not until they're in their 80s or 90s—if they'd take precautions to help reduce their risk of heart disease.

During the past 15 years, medical science has made rapid gains in understanding what causes heart disease. People who have heeded their physician's advice have benefited from the improved awareness. Today's statistics indicate we have a 25% lower rate of heart disease than we did 15 years ago. If we all practiced what research tells us, those figures might be even better.

UNDERSTANDING HOW YOUR HEART WORKS

If you had a vivid picture in your mind of what a heart looks like and could understood how it works, perhaps you would take better care of yours. Imagine your heart is a rubber-bulb syringe about the size of a hand, filled with fluid. Picture your hand holding the rubber-bulb syringe and squeezing down tightly. This forces all the fluid to squirt out. If rubber tubing is attached to the outlet of the syringe, the fluid is forced through the tubing.

Your hand represents the heart muscle. If it is strong and undamaged, it squeezes when your brain instructs your hand to close. In a healthy heart, an automatic electrical impulse causes the muscle cells throughout the heart to contract in an orderly fashion. This automatic contraction pushes the blood inside your heart from chamber to chamber and from the last chamber, the left ventricle, into the blood-vessel system.

The rubber tubing represents your body's blood-vessel system, which is a network of vessels that branches off into smaller vessels until every cell in your body has at least a tiny capillary to supply it with blood that carries oxygen and nourishment and takes away waste products. This network of vessels is estimated to be about 60,000 miles long. Try to imagine a 60,000-mile-long rubber tube attached to the rubber syringe, and you can appreciate how marvelous your heart muscle is. It is only the size of a man's fist, but it pumps life-giving blood to a network more than twice the circumference of the Earth.

It may help to correlate the blood vessels that supply the hand muscle of your imaginary pump to the real heart. At the point where the tube joins the rubber bulb, imagine two branches of tubing veering off and feeding back into the hand muscles. This corresponds to the coronary arteries (tubing branches) and the left heart ventricle (pump), which pumps directly into a large vessel, called the *aorta,* immediately outside the heart.

Coronary arteries branch out of the aorta, go back into the outside of the heart muscle and travel through the muscle called the *myocardium.* These vessels branch out to supply every muscle fiber of the heart with fresh blood, oxygen, potassium, calcium, sodium and glucose. See illustration on page 20.

A heart attack can occur when the heart doesn't beat faithfully. Think about your hand covering the rubber-bulb syringe. Your hand has a blood vessel going into it, which keeps the muscles of your hand strong. If one of the blood vessels supplying your hand becomes blocked or narrowed, part of your hand becomes weakened. If two fingers become weak or dead, your hand can't bend to make a fist. Imagine trying to squeeze that rubber bulb filled with fluid when two fingers can't move. That's what it's like when you have a heart attack. Part of the heart can't squeeze down or force the blood out.

Now imagine the rubber bulb has fluid constantly flowing into it from the other side. If the hand doesn't squeeze all the fluid out, where does it go? First, the bulb will enlarge to accommodate the extra fluid, but it can't get much bigger than it already is. Once the heart enlarges as much as it can, the fluid backs up.

When this happens to a real heart, the heart gets bigger but not stronger. The fluid backs up first into your lungs, making it difficult to breathe, then collects throughout your body. Your liver, abdomen, feet and legs swell, leaving your body weak and fatigued. This condition is called *congestive heart failure.*

Arteriosclerosis is an arterial disease characterized by inelasticity and thickening of the arterial walls, which leads to lessened blood flow. It is commonly called *hardening of the arteries* and can occur anywhere in the body. *Atherosclerosis* is a form of arteriosclerosis in which fatty substances are deposited in and beneath the inner linings of the arterial wall. When vessels of the heart become clogged and blocked by blood clots and other debris, it results in a form of arteriosclerosis called *coronary atherosclerosis.*

Coronary atherosclerosis occurs silently and gradually, sometimes beginning as early as age 15 and certainly by the 20s in many people. If you smoke heavily, eat lots of fatty meat, cheese and butter, and don't exercise, chances are high some vital arteries in your heart will become completely clogged by the time you're 40. This condition is called *coronary artery disease,* and you may suddenly have an un-

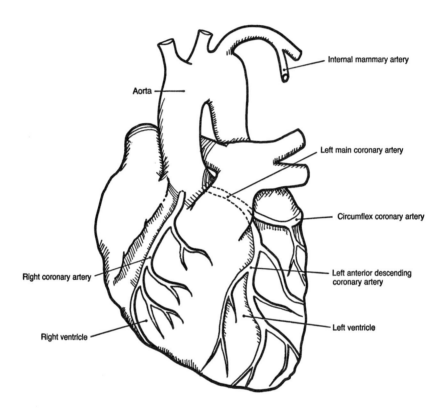

Aorta

Internal mammary artery

Left main coronary artery

Circumflex coronary artery

Right coronary artery

Left anterior descending coronary artery

Left ventricle

Right ventricle

The heart—Right coronary artery branches off from the aorta and nourishes the right side and bottom of the heart. The internal mammary artery lies in the chest wall and may be used to bypass a blocked coronary artery. Left main coronary artery branches into two arteries and nourishes the largest amount of heart muscle; a blockage in this artery can be life-threatening. Left anterior descending coronary artery nourishes the front of the heart, including heart's main pump, the left ventricle. The circumflex coronary artery nourishes the back of the heart. The heart's main pump is the left ventricle, which pumps blood through the aorta (the large blood vessel that carries oxygen-rich blood to your coronary arteries) and the rest of your body.

expected heart attack. Or your heart may be severely weakened from congestive heart failure. Your heart's arteries may be so badly narrowed that every time you do any physical activity or even walk in the cold, you suffer a crushing chest pain—*angina pectoris*—as your heart demands more oxygen.

Let's go back to our bulb-syringe heart. Imagine your hand is squeezing the bulb regularly so fluid flows through the tubing. What happens if the ends of the tube and its branches become clogged and gradually narrow? With the increased resistance, pressure inside the tubing becomes greater, and your hand has to work harder. Eventually, your hand will tire and get weaker. But while your hand is strong enough to work hard, it causes more pressure in the tubing, creating a situation analogous to *high blood pressure.*

It isn't important to our analogy to understand what causes the tubing to clog and narrow—that's complex and many factors are involved. It is important to understand that high blood pressure strains the heart muscle and raises the pressure in vital coronary arteries.

YOU CAN HELP REDUCE YOUR RISKS

Your age, sex and genetic makeup influence your susceptibility to heart disease, and these factors are out of your control. However, many major factors that lead to heart disease *are* within your control. As Paul Dudley White, the father of modern cardiology, said many years ago, "Heart disease before 80 is your own fault." It is a medically accepted fact that daily living habits may determine whether or not you will suffer a heart attack.

If you are overweight, have high blood cholesterol, smoke, do not exercise, drink too much and overreact to regular tensions and stresses in your life, you're a prime candidate for heart disease. But you can change each of these undesirable habits if you're motivated to do so. You *can* beat the odds that they'll strike you down!

In the following sections, you'll learn how risk factors can damage your heart. Take the many risk-factor tests I've included to determine if you're at risk of suffering a heart attack. Then read how you can start right now to help lower your risks and strengthen your heart.

3.

THE MAJOR RISK FACTORS OF HEART DISEASE

*TAKE THIS TEST TO MEASURE YOUR
MAJOR HEART-DISEASE RISKS*

If you scored between *moderate risk* and *very high risk* on the longevity test, page 7, this test will help you pinpoint your risk for heart disease. Circle the score for each characteristic that applies to you. Total the score, then check your risk category beginning on page 27.

Cholesterol

Choose one in each of the following statements.
Your serum cholesterol is:

0	190 or below
+5	191 to 230
+10	231 to 289
+15	290 to 319
+20	Over 320

Your HDL-cholesterol is:

0	Over 60
+5	60 to 45

+10   44 to 36
+15   35 to 28
+20   27 to 22

In your family:
  0   There is no history of abnormally elevated cholesterol in a close relative
+1   One parent, aunt, uncle or grandparent had an abnormally high cholesterol level
+2   Two parents, aunts, uncles or grandparents had an abnormally high cholesterol level
+3   More than two close relatives had an abnormally high cholesterol level

You exercise vigorously for at least 1/2 hour:
 -3   Almost every day
 -2   Several times a week
+2   Only on weekends
+5   Only occasionally, if at all

You eat beef, pork, cold cuts, lamb or sausage:
  0   Less than once a week
+1   Once a week
+2   Twice a week
+3   More than 3 times a week
+4   More than 3 times a week, and your cholesterol level is above 220

You eat eggs:
  0   Rarely
+1   1 or 2 a week, alone or in prepared food
+2   3 or 4 a week, alone or in prepared food
+3   5 or 6 a week, alone or in prepared food
+4   5 or more a week, and your cholesterol level is above 220

You use butter (not margarine):
  0   Rarely
+1   Every day on bread
+2   Every day on bread and vegetables
+3   Every day on bread and vegetables and in cooking

You eat ice cream:
   0   Rarely
  +2   About once a week
  +3   Several times a week
  +4   Usually every day

You drink milk:
   0   Usually skim milk, every day
  +1   Usually 1% fat milk, every day
  +2   Usually 2% fat milk, every day
  +4   Usually whole milk, every day

You eat cheese (except low-fat cottage cheese):
   0   Rarely
  +1   Once a week
  +2   Twice a week
  +3   3 times a week
  +4   More than 3 times a week

In cooking you use:
  −2   Corn, sesame, safflower or olive oil
  −1   Soybean oil
   0   Solid vegetable shortening or margarine
  +4   Coconut or palm oil or butter

You eat cold-water, fatty fish, such as salmon, tuna (fresh or water-packed), halibut, mackerel, trout:
  −3   At least 4 or 5 times a week
  −2   2 or 3 times a week
  −1   Once a week
   0   Rarely

You eat cake, cookies, pastries:
   0   Rarely
  +1   Once a week
  +2   2 or 3 times a week
  +3   Almost every day

Smoking

Choose one in each of the following statements.
Your cigarette-smoking history is:

  0   Never smoked, or quit over 5 years ago
+3   Quit 1 to 5 years ago
+6   Quit during the past year

The number of cigarettes you currently smoke is:

 +9   1/2 to 1 pack a day
+12   1 to 2 packs a day
+15   More than 2 packs a day

You have smoked cigarettes:

  0   Never smoked, or quit over 5 years ago
 +1   Only for the last year
 +2   For last 5 years
 +3   For last 10 years
 +4   For 10 to 20 years
+10   For more than 20 years and began as an adult
+15   For more than 20 years and began as a teenager

The quality of the air you breathe is:

  0   Unpolluted by smoke, exhaust or industry at home *and* at work
+2   Unpolluted, except you live *or* work with smokers
+4   Unpolluted, except you live *and* work with smokers
+6   Polluted at work or home, and you live *or* work with smokers
+8   Polluted at work or home, and you live *and* work with smokers

Blood Pressure

Choose one in each of the following statements.
Your blood pressure is:

  0   Below 120/75
 +2   120/75 to 140/85
 +6   140/85 to 150/90
 +8   150/90 to 175/100
+10   175/100 to 190/110
+12   Above 190/110

In your family:
- 0   No history of high blood pressure in a close relative
- +1   One parent, aunt, uncle or grandparent had high blood pressure
- +2   Two parents, aunts, uncles or grandparents had high blood pressure
- +3   More than two close relatives had high blood pressure

You salt your food:
- −2   Never or rarely add salt
- +1   During cooking but not at the table
- +2   Taste food and often add salt
- +3   At the table before tasting it
- +6   At the table and have blood pressure over 120/75

You exercise (even if no more vigorously than a long walk) for at least 1/2 hour:
- −3   Almost every day
- −2   Several times a week
- −1   Only on weekends
- +3   Only occasionally, if at all
- +4   Rarely exercise and have blood pressure over 140/90

You react to stress at home or work by:
- −2   Talking about your problems to a friend or loved one then taking action to try to correct the situation
- +1   Worrying about the problem then taking action to correct the situation
- +2   Worrying about the problem but doing nothing about it because you feel helpless
- +3   Getting angry and losing your temper
- +4   Getting angry but concealing your feelings
- +6   Getting angry or frustrated, and your blood pressure is over 140/90

Calculating Your Score

Take your scores for each category, and rescore them as shown below:

Cholesterol	**Smoking**	**Blood Pressure**
50 to 80 = 7	26 to 44 = 5	23 to 32 = 5
40 to 49 = 6	16 to 25 = 4	16 to 22 = 4
30 to 39 = 5	11 to 15 = 3	11 to 15 = 3
20 to 29 = 4	4 to 10 = 2	4 to 10 = 2
13 to 19 = 3	−7 to 3 = 1	0 to 3 = 1
7 to 12 = 2		
−5 to 6 = 1		

Fill in your scores below, then multiply them together to determine your final score.

_____ X _____ X _____ = _____
  Cholesterol   Smoking   Blood Pressure   Total

INTERPRETING YOUR SCORE

Check your total score below to see if your health and your life are at risk. You may be referred to the risk-reducing nutrition plan, page 186, or the risk-reducing exercise plan, page 226.

1 to 26   **Low Risk**—Your risk of heart disease is not due to elevated cholesterol, high blood pressure or cigarette smoking. A score of less than 20 indicates a minimal risk of heart disease. A score over 20 means a poor family history, and many minor risk factors probably combine to give you a slightly elevated risk of heart disease. Take the risk-factor test that begins on page 37 to see if you can lower some of your risks.

27 to 124   **Moderate Risk**—Though your cholesterol level and blood pressure are not alarmingly high, and you may smoke only a little, if at all, the combined effect puts you at a moderate risk of heart disease. Study the test to see where you earned points, then take action to eliminate those risk factors by following the risk-reducing nutrition plan and the risk-reducing exercise plan.

125 to 139   **High Risk**—The combined effects of smoking, eating a high-fat diet and elevated cholesterol are putting you at high risk of heart disease. Begin to change your ways *now* if you want to help protect yourself from a heart attack. Stop smoking, and follow the risk-reducing nutrition plan and the risk-reducing exercise plan outlined in this book.

140 +   **Very High Risk**—All your habits are excessive and put you at very high risk of heart disease. If you change your diet, lower your blood pressure and stop smoking, you may lower your risk. Follow the risk-reducing nutrition plan and the risk-reducing exercise plan to help lower your risks.

The Major Risk Factors of Heart Disease

You can prevent yourself from being a victim of heart disease—even if you have a family history of it. Science has shown that your lifestyle plays a part in causing atherosclerosis, one form of heart disease. A number of large-scale, long-term studies carried out by medical researchers all point the finger at the same causes:

- A high serum-cholesterol level.
- High blood pressure.
- Cigarette smoking.

The most well-known study began in 1948 in Framingham, Massachusetts, and data is still being collected today from the same community. Researchers chose this community because it represented a cross section of people. This research study, directed by Dr. William Kannel of Boston University and Dr. William Castelli of Harvard University, collects medical data every 2 years from more than 5,000 people between the ages of 30 and 60. Each participant is profiled thoroughly, and almost every conceivable type of information is collected and stored in a large data bank. Numerous small studies evaluate the data, weighing separate and multiple risk factors.

Many other studies from prominent research institutions, such as the National Heart, Lung and Blood Institute, the University of Michigan, Northwestern University and the University of Chicago, have reached many of the same conclusions.

THE CHOLESTEROL RISK FACTOR

Your blood contains a group of fatty substances called *lipids*. Several of these lipids—cholesterol, low-density lipoproteins and triglycerides—can be harmful to your body. When they exist in your blood in excessive amounts, they appear to be related to the process of atherosclerosis. Cholesterol is the fatty substance that we are most concerned about.

The association between cholesterol and heart disease was discovered around the turn of the century when pathologists examined blood vessels of victims who had died of heart-attacks and/or vascular disease. Pathologists discovered these victims' vessels were clogged with a mushy, yellow substance that slowed the blood flow, and blood vessels were often hardened and calcified. Further studies revealed the predominant substance in the mush was cholesterol. Since then, scientists have debated the exact role cholesterol plays in vascular disease, but many do not doubt that cholesterol plays a major role. Most scientists investigating atherosclerosis see cholesterol as playing a pivotal role in the development of the disease.

A report of a 10-year study, headed by Dr. Basil Rifkind of the Lipid Research Clinics at the National Heart, Lung and Blood Institute in Bethesda, Maryland, dramatically demonstrated the correlation between serum-cholesterol levels and heart disease. This well-designed experiment followed nearly 4,000 men for 7 to 10 years. Some men in the group had their serum cholesterol lowered by a special diet; others achieved lower cholesterol levels by a combination of diet and drug therapy. The group treated with diet and drug therapy had a 24% reduction in death from coronary disease and a 19% lower risk of non-fatal heart attacks than men in the control group who made no efforts to lower their cholesterol.

In the 1940s, an experiment done by Forest Kendall and Alfred Steiner at Columbia University produced coronary atherosclerosis in dogs by feeding them large quantities of egg yolk, which is high in cholesterol. Since then, thousands of studies have been conducted to determine why cholesterol-containing blockages develop and to determine what can be done about them. There are many theories, but there is *no consensus* as to why cholesterol builds up in arteries. Almost without exception, leading heart specialists, pathologists and medical investigators now agree that excess cholesterol in the blood is related to diet. Despite controversy over details, it may be a good idea to choose foods that are lower in cholesterol content. Clogging of arteries can begin as early as age 15 or 20, so there's no time to lose in preventing cholesterol buildup.

The lower your serum-cholesterol level, the lower the risk of atherosclerosis, but there's more to it than that. The cholesterol molecule consists of several varieties of lipoprotein. These lipoproteins are named according to their density when spun in a centrifuge—very low- (VLDL), low- (LDL), intermediate- (IDL) and high-density- (HDL) lipoprotein.

It appears the higher the LDL and the lower the HDL in the makeup of the total serum cholesterol, the greater the likelihood of being stricken with coronary heart disease. The risk is lower if there is less LDL and more HDL because LDL appears to deposit cholesteral in the arteries, and HDL flushes it out. Several recent studies indicate a blood substance called *apolipoprotein* (A1) may be the most accurate predictor of a person's potential for developing coronary artery disease. As of now, there is no test available for use by ordinary medical laboratories to test for A1, but one may be available in the near future. The high-density lipoprotein group also contains two or three different lipoprotein components (fractions); these are also under intense study to find out which ones are associated with a decreased risk of coronary heart disease.

When you go to your doctor for a checkup, ask for a cholesterol count and a reading of your LDL and HDL levels.

Cholesterol levels in the blood can range from a very healthy 120 mg/dl to an unhealthy 380 mg/dl. (Mg/dl is a measurement of milligrams per deciliter.) Levels above 380 are seriously abnormal because of an unusual hereditary condition and may put you at perilous risk of heart attack. Specialized treatment, including cholesterol-lowering drugs, are needed to control abnormal cholesterol levels.

HDL cholesterol ranges from a very healthy high (the higher the better compared to the total cholesterol level) of 80 mg/dl to a risky low of 20 mg/dl. The HDL/cholesterol ratio can be determined by dividing the HDL level into the total cholesterol level. For example, if you have an HDL of 40 and a total cholesterol of 200, you have a ratio of 1 to 5. A ratio of 1 to 5 or higher in a male indicates some risk of having a heart attack. An even higher ratio (1 to between 6 and 10) may mean a greater likelihood of heart attack, especially if other heart-disease risk factors are present. The best situation to have is high HDL, 60 or above, and low cholesterol, about 150, for a ratio closer to 2.

Until recently, medical researchers believed a cholesterol level of 200 was adequate for protection from heart disease. Research from the Lipid-Metabolism-Atherogenisis branch of the National Heart, Lung and Blood Institute indicates lower levels, such as 150, may decrease risks when compared to a level of 200.

You can improve your HDL/cholesterol ratio by elevating your HDL and lowering your total cholesterol. A low-fat, low-cholesterol diet, regular exercise, not smoking, moderate use of alcohol and weight loss accomplishes both goals.

I give you more information about nutrition in the section that begins on page 186. The nutrition plan restricts fatty meats, organ meats, chicken and duck skin, butter, egg yolks, cheeses and dairy fat.

Exercise has also been shown by many studies to lower cholesterol levels. If you lead a sedentary life, find some way to include aerobic exercises in your daily activities. I provide you with information and guidance on how to exercise in the section that begins on page 226. Follow the risk-reducing exercise plan, and you'll help exercise your way to good health.

Triglycerides, which are large molecules of fat found in the bloodstream, can also increase your risk of heart disease. Dietary fat is transported from the intestines to the liver in the form of triglycerides. It can take as long as 12 to 14 hours to clear them from the bloodstream. A high serum-triglyceride level has been correlated with a risk of heart disease. Triglyceride levels are invariably low when HDL-cholesterol levels are high. A blood test for triglycerides is not routinely necessary, but a test should be done at least once.

A malfunctioning liver may deposit triglycerides in the bloodstream. Excess alcohol consumption induces the liver to manufacture abnormal amounts of triglycerides and hinders the clearance of triglycerides from the blood, which may increase your risk of heart disease.

If a triglyceride blood test is necessary, you must fast for 14 hours before the test. This clears out triglycerides that come from your diet. Only then can an accurate measure be made of triglycerides that are the result of excess fat in the diet or a malfunctioning liver. A normal triglyceride level after a 14-hour period of not eating should be below 150 mg/dl. If it is more than 300 mg/dl, the HDL will be very low, and specialized medical care is necessary.

THE CIGARETTE RISK FACTOR

Another major risk factor for heart disease is cigarette smoking. Cigarette smoking damages your cardiovascular system; when you smoke, your blood pressure rises, your HDL cholesterol goes down, blood platelets (the blood's clotting cells) become stickier, your heart rate speeds up and abnormal heartbeats occur more often.

Smoking reduces the oxygen-carrying capacity of your red blood cells because cigarette smoke contains carbon monoxide. You suck this poisonous gas into your lungs, and it competes with oxygen for a place on the hemoglobin molecule. Carbon monoxide latches onto the red blood cells in place of oxygen. Rushing through your bloodstream, carbon monoxide reduces the availability of oxygen to your heart muscle, brain and other vital organs—not without ill effect. People who smoke have about 20% less oxygen in their blood than non-smokers!

Nicotine is also absorbed into your bloodstream; one of its effects is to stimulate the release of the hormone adrenalin. Adrenalin is a central-nervous-system stimulant that causes many effects. Your heart beats more rapidly, your blood pressure rises, your blood vessels become constricted and your blood clots more readily when adrenalin is released in the body. Your speeded up heart and body require more oxygen, but because of the carbon monoxide in your blood, you have less oxygen than your body needs.

Pipe smokers absorb as much nicotine as cigarette smokers, but they do not have significantly higher rates of heart disease than non-smokers. Pipe smokers don't usually inhale, so researchers have concluded that the combination of inhaled nicotine and carbon monoxide probably does the greatest damage to the heart muscle.

A single cigarette reduces your heart's stroke volume (the amount of blood pumped with each beat), increases the frequency of abnormal beats, raises your blood pressure and speeds up your pulse. Smoking one pack of cigarettes a day *triples* the risk of death from coronary heart disease compared to the risk for a non-smoker.

Smokers have more atherosclerosis in their coronary arteries, a higher incidence of heart attacks and a greater chance of dying suddenly from a heart attack than non-smokers. The younger a person is when he starts smoking, the more likely he is to be a lifelong smoker, the deeper he is likely to inhale and the younger he is likely to die! If you stop smoking, your risk of heart disease is lowered significantly.

If you smoke low-tar, low-nicotine cigarettes, don't fool yourself into thinking you're safe. Studies by Dr. E. Hammond of the American Cancer Society show people who switch to these types of cigarettes unconsciously inhale more deeply and smoke more cigarettes to obtain the same amount of nicotine as they got from high-nicotine cigarettes. They may be doing themselves more harm because they are getting more carbon monoxide.

Cigarette smoking is not only an independent risk factor; it *multiplies* the risks already present from high cholesterol and high blood pressure. If you smoke and have a high cholesterol level, you're compounding your risk 4 times. Younger men and women who smoke have a considerably higher risk of heart disease than those who do not.

Women who take birth-control pills and smoke are at higher risk of heart attack and stroke than women who do not smoke or take birth-control pills. Doctors generally recommend women in this situation stop the pill, especially if they are over 35, or stop smoking.

If you stop smoking now, your damaged cardiovascular system—and lungs—will begin to repair themselves. It takes 5 years before repair is achieved, but your system can return to the healthy state of a non-smoker.

Many scientific studies bear this out. A study reported in the *British Heart Journal,* which followed a group of male smokers (age 45 to 64) for 18 years, showed those who stopped smoking had a heart-attack rate that was half that of men in the study who continued to smoke.

Another study followed 100 male heart-attack victims who were 45 or under who smoked. Within 1 year of the heart attack, none of those who quit smoking had another heart attack, but 17% of those who continued to smoke did. After 3 years, still none of those who quit had a recurrence, but 52% of the smokers had suffered another heart attack!

I believe many, if not most, people who smoke would like to stop—they simply don't know how. If you're a smoker, I hope these frightening facts will give you the incentive to do something to stop smoking. It's difficult for most people to do it on their own because cigarette smoking is a drug addiction—an addiction to nicotine— and quitting involves suffering unpleasant side effects.

If you can't do it on your own, join a stop-smoking program, such as those offered by the American Cancer Society or the American Heart Association. These groups are highly effective and give you the needed moral support to kick the habit.

If you are a non-smoker, don't automatically feel free of risk. Dr. W. S. Aranson reported in the *New England Journal of Medicine* that people who do not smoke but who live or work with heavy smokers develop heart disease (and cancer) more readily. A non-smoking person with heart trouble can suffer angina pectoris pains if he breathes air polluted with cigarette smoke (or car exhaust) because he is breathing air heavily polluted with carbon monoxide.

The extent of the harm caused by *passive smoke* (smoke from others' cigarettes) is still being debated, but there is agreement that it's dangerous to your health. Do everything in your power to encourage those around you to stop smoking and clean up the air!

THE HYPERTENSION RISK FACTOR

Another major risk factor in heart disease is hypertension, also called *high blood pressure.* Thirty-seven million people who live in the United States have hypertension. It is particularly dangerous because its harmful effects on your body occur without you knowing anything is wrong. That's why it's called the *silent killer.* Symptoms may not be apparent, but the damage can be fatal if it is ignored.

Blood pressure, weight and smoking habits of students entering the University of Pennsylvania and Harvard University were recorded several decades ago and recently analyzed by Dr. Ralph Paffenberger of Harvard University. Analysis showed that elevated blood pressure at the time the student entered college indicated a risk of coronary heart disease 20, 30 and even 40 years later.

Your doctor measures your blood pressure by taking an indirect reading. He wraps a cuff around your arm just above the elbow, where a large artery comes close to the surface. The cuff tightens around your arm as air is pumped into it. The doctor reads the amount of pressure put into the cuff in millimeters of mercury on a manometer. As he reduces the air pressure in the cuff, he listens with a stethoscope for your pulse to return in the closed-off artery. When he hears the pulse come through, he reads the manometer. This reading is the *systolic blood pressure,* the pressure when the heart contracts. Slowly reducing the air pressure in the cuff from that point until the pulse sound disappears determines the *diastolic blood pressure,* the pressure when the heart is at rest.

Your pulse corresponds to each beat of your heart. The systolic level represents the pressure at the end of each heartbeat contraction and corresponds to the closing of your fist in our imaginary bulb-syringe heart. The diastolic reading represents the pressure as the heart relaxes before the next beat, which corresponds to the opening of your fist.

Normal blood pressure usually varies from moment to moment, depending on your degree of physical and mental relaxation. It increases with exertion and anxiety. If your doctor suspects your blood pressure is abnormally high, readings will be taken at several different times when you are as relaxed as possible.

The lower the systolic pressure, the better—if you are healthy. Doctors consider readings even as low as 90 healthy. A low systolic blood pressure has nothing to do with being tired or sluggish, as some people believe. One can be an Olympic champion with a blood pressure of 90/60.

The diastolic blood pressure has a normal range of 60 to 85mm Hg (milligrams of mercury). The lower the pressure, the better. The best blood pressure at any age would be a systolic between 90 and 120 and a diastolic of 60 to 75mm Hg. A reading of 130/80 is acceptable, but above 140/90 is considered mildly elevated.

It is normal—but not necessarily desirable—for your blood pressure to increase as you get older. As you age, your vascular system develops a mild rigidity and less elasticity in the walls of the arteries. This is the early stage of hardening of the arteries.

This change causes the systolic pressure to go up more than the diastolic, so a reading of 150/90 could be reasonable if you are over 60. This is acceptable and does not require medication.

Generally, doctors allow for an increase in the systolic reading of up to 140mm Hg to age 50. Perhaps 150 or even 160mm Hg would be acceptable for someone over 65. But such levels are *not ideal* and are an avoidable part of aging.

There is a popular misconception that the "lower number" (diastolic) is the only one that counts. This is *not* true. Systolic hypertension carries with it every risk that diastolic hypertension does—if not more! This is especially true of the elderly, in whom systolic hypertension is quite common.

Symptoms of high blood pressure may not be apparent, but damage can be fatal if it is ignored. It's as if a motor were pumping water through a hose that has the far end closed off—the motor keeps pumping against this unnaturally high pressure. This is the way the heart works in a person with high blood pressure. The heart must pump over 100,000 beats a day against greater pressure than it is intended to handle. Along with the heart, the kidneys and brain can also be damaged.

Labile hypertension, a condition in which your blood pressure is high on one occasion and later found to be normal, should not be ignored. It is also a risk factor. Be sure your blood pressure is taken accurately and varying readings aren't due to faulty technique or equipment. The electronic units found in shopping centers are not as accurate as they should be. Your physician is more reliable.

Several studies bear out the importance of labile hypertension. The Framingham 18-year follow-up study showed people whose blood pressure was occasionally only modestly above normal carried a 40% greater risk of getting cardiovascular disease than those whose blood pressure was *always* normal.

It's best to take an average of several pressure readings at random in a doctor's office to determine whether or not your blood pressure requires correction by drugs. One high reading shouldn't label you hypertensive, but it should not be ignored because a condition of labile hypertension is not without risk.

Excessive dietary sodium can also raise blood pressure in susceptible people. The most common ways people ingest sodium is through table salt and sodium used in food processing. Though sodium is a necessary mineral needed to keep your body functioning, it's unhealthy to have too much of it. You get sufficient sodium from a balanced diet without salt added during cooking or at the table. But our modern diet of fast-food, packaged food and prepared food is loaded with excess sodium.

Some people can consume excess sodium without having it cause hypertension, but unfortunately there is no way of predicting who is susceptible and who is not. If you can't reduce excess salt or eliminate packaged and processed foods from your diet, have your blood pressure checked regularly. As long as it remains at a safe level, sodium probably does little harm. But if you develop even slightly elevated blood pressure, cut out the sodium.

Often all that needs to be done to control mild hypertension is to go on a low-sodium, high-potassium, high-calcium diet. This means you must prepare all foods without adding salt, avoid highly salted foods, such as crackers, nuts and pickles, and eliminate many processed foods, such as puddings, ketchup, cheese and canned foods, from your diet. Check labels for sodium content. The responsibility of following this diet is with you—you can control this risk factor.

Your doctor may prescribe a diuretic drug to help your body excrete excess water and sodium. It's important that other important minerals, such as potassium and magnesium, aren't excreted in excess along with the extra sodium. Your doctor should take periodic blood tests and will prescribe supplements if this becomes a problem.

As a general rule, mild-to-moderate hypertension can be controlled by implementing the following measures:

● Follow a diet low in sodium and high in potassium and calcium.

● Lose weight, if necessary.

● Exercise regularly.

● Relax periodically throughout the day.

● Control your reactions to stress.

● Drink no more than moderate amounts of alcohol (less than 3 ounces of hard liquor no more than 5 days a week).

The major risk factors of heart disease are a matter of lifestyle, and they are within your control. If you're serious about beating the odds of getting heart disease, you *can* make a difference.

4.

THE (NOT-SO) MINOR
RISKS OF HEART DISEASE

*TAKE THIS TEST TO MEASURE YOUR
(NOT-SO) MINOR HEART-DISEASE RISKS*

This test measures the *cumulative effect* of other risk factors of heart disease—small risks that when combined may equal a big risk! Circle the score for each characteristic that applies to you. Total the score, then check your risk category on page 41.

Personal

Choose one.

You are a:

- 0   Woman younger than 55
- +1   Man younger than 55
- +2   Woman 55 or older
- +3   Man 55 to 65
- +4   Man 66 or older

Weight

Choose one in each of the following statements.

Your present weight is:

0   Within 10% of ideal
+1   More than 20% overweight
+2   More than 30% overweight
+3   More than 40% overweight

During the course of your adult life, your weight has fluctuated from your present weight by:

+1   10 pounds up or down
+2   20 pounds up or down
+3   30 pounds or more, up or down

You began to be overweight during:

+1   Your 30s
+2   Your 20s
+3   Childhood or adolescence

You have gone on a fad diet:

+1   Several times in your life
+2   About once a year during past several years or longer
+3   More than once a year during past several years or longer

Alcohol and Drug Consumption

Choose one in each of the following statements.

You drink alcoholic beverages:

0   Never, or only socially (less than once a month)
+1   Only one 5-ounce glass of wine or one 12-ounce glass of beer or 1-1/2 ounces of liquor about 5 times a week
+2   Two 5-ounce glasses of wine or two 12-ounce glasses of beer or 3 ounces of liquor about 5 times a week
+4   More than 3 ounces of liquor or more than three 5-ounce glasses of wine or three 12-ounce glasses of beer almost every day

You take diet pills or amphetamines:

+2   3 times a week
+4   4 to 7 times a week
+6   3 or more times a week and also have high blood pressure or elevated cholesterol

You use birth-control pills, and you are:

+2 Over 35 and do not smoke
+3 Under 35 and smoke
+5 Over 35 and smoke

You are post-menopausal, and you have taken estrogen for:

+1 5 years or less
+2 5 to 10 years
+3 More than 10 years

Diabetes

Choose one.

Your blood-sugar tolerance is:

 0 Completely normal and always has been
+1 Slightly elevated glucose (prediabetic) or low (hypoglycemic), and you are a woman
+2 Slightly elevated (prediabetic) or low (hypoglycemic), and you are a man
+3 Diabetic not requiring insulin or drug control
+4 Diabetic after age 40 requiring strict dietary or insulin or drug control
+5 Diabetic before age 30 requiring strict dietary or insulin or drug control

Exercise

Choose one in each of the following statements.

During the day your job or occupation involves:

-3 Almost continual, heavy, physical work
-2 Constant, though not demanding, physical work
+1 A little physical activity
+3 Almost no physical activity; you sit most of the day

You exercise during your occupation or leisure time:

-3 Almost every day
-2 5 times a week
-1 2 or 3 times a week
+1 Only on weekends
+4 Rarely or not at all

While you exercise you:
- −3   Work up a heavy sweat and breathe deeply
- −2   Work up a light sweat and breathe moderately
- 0   Do not sweat or breathe any harder than usual
- +3   You do not exercise

Each time you exercise you spend:
- −3   1/2 hour or more
- −2   20 minutes to 1/2 hour
- 0   10 to 15 minutes
- +3   You do not exercise

You have been exercising:
- −3   All your life
- −2   For the past 5 years or more
- −1   For the past 2 years
- +3   Have always been inactive or have been during adulthood

Stress

Choose one in each of the following statements.
Your marriage, home and family life are:
- 0   Pleasant and satisfying
- +1   Satisfying but there are often disagreements
- +2   Unsatisfying with frequent heated disagreements
- +3   Stressful with openly hostile relationships

Your job or occupation is:
- 0   Rewarding and often demanding
- +1   Unrewarding and demanding
- +2   Unrewarding and not demanding
- +3   Unrewarding and often very frustrating

You feel depressed, have a headache or insomnia, are constipated or have diarrhea or indigestion:
- 0   Rarely or not at all
- +1   Once in awhile
- +2   More than once a week
- +3   Several times a week
- +4   Daily

INTERPRETING YOUR SCORE

To determine your score, add all scores from the categories. Check the total score below to see if your health and your life are at risk.

-15 to 8   **Low Risk**—Your weight, exercise habits and lifestyle are excellent to very good. Keep it up, and you shouldn't have to worry about the not-so-minor risk factors compounding your risk of heart disease. If you scored at risk on the risk-factor test on page 22, you still have some changes to make.

9 to 26   **Moderate Risk**—You are at moderate risk from risk factors causing heart attacks. You probably need to lose weight and exercise more to lower your risk of heart disease. If you scored at risk on the risk-factor test on page 22, you still have some changes to make.

27 to 40   **High Risk**—You are at high risk of suffering a heart attack due to the risk factors discussed in this section. The less-significant risk factors of heart disease are combining to put your health in jeopardy. If you scored high on the risk-factor test on page 22, you may be at serious risk. Study the test to see where you scored a 2 or 3, then make an effort to eliminate them to help lower your risk of heart disease.

41+   **Very High Risk**—All the not-so-minor risk factors of heart disease are working together to create one large risk! When combined with other risks, you may have a serious health problem. You can help lower your risk by taking seriously the advice I offer in this book, but you have little time to waste!

The (Not-So) Minor Risks of Heart Disease

High cholesterol, high blood pressure and cigarette smoking are the leading causes of heart disease. Other less-serious—but not to be ignored—risk factors also compound the seriousness of the problem. Poor physical condition, overweight, excessive alcohol consumption and stress are each risk factors for developing heart disease. When several of these conditions exist together, your risk may be compounded significantly!

It makes sense to eliminate as many risk factors from your personal life as you can. Eliminating some risks may require breaking bad or lazy habits, such as losing weight or reducing your alcohol consumption. Eliminating other risks may mean a significant change in your lifestyle. The choice is yours.

YOUR PHYSICAL CONDITION MAY AFFECT YOUR RISK

Many studies show extremely active people have a lower heart-attack rate than those who are sedentary. It's an accepted fact that if you don't include regular physical activity in your life, your risk of developing heart disease is greater.

If you're active, you have a better chance of surviving a heart attack than if you are sedentary. You have a lower chance of dying suddenly, and you're less likely to acquire many forms of serious illness during middle age.

Your body is a complex machine, built for motion. It functions best when exercised regularly, at a vigorous pace. Exercise plays a major role in achieving an optimally functioning body. Without exercise, you can't achieve the sense of well-being you need to be energetic, confident and poised. You may be subject to a range of ailments that might otherwise be avoidable, such as hypertension, coronary disease, ulcers, diabetes, low-back pain, emotionally induced tension states, less adaptability to stress and lower levels of mental alertness. Exercise puts more life into your years and more years onto your life.

Several well-controlled scientific studies support the conclusion that to be physically inactive is dangerous to your health. A study performed at the Stanford University Medical Center by Dr. Ralph Paffenberger followed 17,000 Harvard alumni men for up to 10 years. Another study, published in the *New England Journal of Medicine,* followed 12,000 San Francisco longshoremen over many years. These studies compared vigorously active, moderately active and inactive men between the ages of 35 and 74. Conclusions showed a convincing *doubled risk* of heart attack and a *tripled risk* of sudden death from heart attack among men in the low-activity category when compared to those in the high-activity category.

Vigorous exercise provided the greatest protection. The study of Harvard graduates showed if an individual increased his physical activity to a high level, he could lower his risk of coronary heart disease by 25%. If he only stopped smoking, the risk was also lowered by 25%. If only high blood pressure was lowered, the risk was lessened by 16%. Combining increased exercise with not smoking reduced the risks of heart disease by 30%.

Another large study done in New York of 55,000 men, aged 25 to 64, showed when heart attacks occurred, attacks were 3 times more likely to be fatal in sedentary men than in active men.

In Britain, an 8-year-long study of 18,000 civil-service workers carried out by Dr. Jerry Morris and published in the medical journal *Lancet* showed that vigorous exercise only on *weekends* gave a benefit of 50% fewer heart problems. This benefit occurred at all ages. Exercise was particularly beneficial for men in their 70s, despite the presence of other coronary risk factors.

It's better to exercise more often than just on weekends. It's safer for the heart and more beneficial for true conditioning if you begin and continue a *regular* exercise program.

A sedentary life also encourages physiologic deteriorations that cause aging to proceed more rapidly. Circulation to vital organs slows, and tiny capillaries close, reducing the effectiveness of your brain, heart, lungs, spinal cord, nerves, muscles and other vital organs. Exercise is necessary to keep capillaries open and circulation healthy.

If your father or mother died prematurely of coronary disease and did not smoke, did not drink heavily or was not obese, you may be afflicted with the same *potential*. I use the word "prematurely" because the difference between a genetic cause of the disease and one acquired through poor living habits is not similar in its effect on you—unless you "inherited" the same unhealthy lifestyle. Other factors, such as diabetes, high blood pressure and a personality that reacts strongly to stress, may also be at the root of early heart disease.

Anyone who has a family history of premature heart disease should be diligent in eliminating all other risk factors. If you lower your risk factors, your genetic predisposition may never manifest itself.

Another factor that affects your risk of developing heart disease is overweight. Excess weight can lead to hypertension, hyperlipidemia, diabetes, angina pectoris, heart failure and even sudden death. Overweight can compound your risk of heart disease if you have other risk factors. If you are obese (more than 20% overweight), it *is* cause for concern, especially if you are under 50. Obese men can expect to live 20% shorter lives and obese women 10% shorter lives than their normal-weight counterparts.

Many doctors believe obesity causes adult-onset diabetes, but this has not been scientifically proven. Diabetes is 5 times more prevalent in obese people over age 40 than it is in lean people in the same age group. About 80% of the people who suffer from adult-onset, non-insulin dependent diabetes are also overweight.

Diabetes enhances and quickens the process of hardening of the arteries throughout the body, such as the heart, kidneys and brain. You *must* try to keep your weight under control. In the section that begins on page 204, I describe how you can lose weight permanently, without risk, by following my weight-reduction plan.

Several years ago, medical investigators studying blood pressure and cardiovascular disease noted in areas where the drinking water was hard people had lower rates of heart disease and hypertension than in areas where water was soft.

Researchers do not understand the reason for this because hard water does not effect cholesterol levels, and the amount of sodium in the water seems to play no significant role. But hard water has more dissolved minerals in it than soft water, and some researchers believe the calcium and magnesium found in the water, which are needed for a healthy heart and blood vessels, might be the key.

A deficiency in calcium is an important factor in high blood pressure. People who drink hard water are less likely to be deficient in calcium. Those who drink soft water get less calcium from their drinking water, perhaps explaining their significantly higher incidence of hypertension. Artificially softened water is excessively high in sodium.

This theory has not been confirmed, but if you drink soft water, make sure you get adequate amounts of calcium and other minerals in your diet. If you live in a hard-water area and your water is artificially softened, be sure the water you drink is untreated. That way you'll avoid ingesting unnecessary sodium.

THE ALCOHOL RISK FACTOR

Overindulgence in alcohol gradually poisons your heart muscles. It can destroy the heart just as it does the liver, brain and other vital organs. Most people aren't aware of this risk, but doctors who treat heavy drinkers, especially younger people who began drinking heavily in their teens, see the condition frequently.

If you begin to drink heavily later in life, you are more likely to die of brain hemorrhage caused by the hypertensive effect of alcohol rather than from an alcohol-induced heart condition.

Heavy drinkers—whether they drink wine, beer or hard liquor—have a higher incidence of heart attack than moderate or non-drinkers. Heavy drinking can cause muscle-power failure or a breakdown of electrical-nerve impulses. Alcohol harms your heart in two ways.

- It can damage the muscles.
- It can damage nerves needed to stimulate the muscles to contract and pump blood.

Your heart can be damaged by years of excessive alcohol consumption. Muscles can be damaged to such a degree that they become swollen with fluid and contract ineffectively, causing the heart to become large, dilated and flabby. This condition is called *alcoholic cardiomyopathy*. It is usually irreversible and eventually results in death due to congestive failure, embolism or sudden death.

Another effect alcohol can have on your heart is to interfere with the normal heartbeat. This disruption of the heart's electrical system, called *arrhythmias*, manifests itself in many ways; some are fatal. A total disruption of the heart's orderly impulse system can occur, causing *atrial fibrillation,* which can lead to stroke and other problems that can kill you.

Years of heavy drinking can cause these conditions, but people who don't usually drink heavily can die suddenly after consuming a large amount of alcohol. Autopsies show no other apparent causes of death except damage to the heart's electrical system. Every year, hospital emergency rooms across the country experience a notable increase in the number of patients admitted with cardiac arrhythmias at Christmas and New Year's—due to the tradition of celebrating the holidays with liberal amounts of alcohol. They call this the *holiday heart syndrome,* and it is no cause for celebration.

The cardiac reaction to alcohol is reversible once the heart's rhythm is restored if the victim abstains from excessive amounts of alcohol. Unfortunately, it is not always apparent that a heart rhythm irregularity is present until it has progressed to a more serious stage.

Don't be fooled into thinking you aren't at risk of developing these conditions because I use the word "overindulgence" to describe how much alcohol poisons the heart. Most of us consider our own behavior normal and behavior that differs from ours as "abnormal." If put on the spot, most heavy drinkers define their own habits as moderate and those of people who drink more than they do as excessive—no matter how much they actually drink. They probably believe what they're saying.

It *is* safe to drink moderately. "Moderately" is defined as drinking only 4 or 5 days a week; each day you consume no more than two 5-ounce glasses of wine or two 12-ounce glasses of beer or no more than two cocktails containing a *total* of 3 ounces of hard liquor. I tell my patients any more alcohol than this on a regular basis can cause heart damage and high blood pressure, as well as liver cirrhosis. Even "moderate" consumption is being defined more critically by a few researchers—they believe an even lower intake of alcohol is more moderate.

Some researchers believe moderate use of alcohol may protect you from heart disease by stimulating the liver to produce high-density lipoprotein cholesterol (HDL), which has a protective effect against the development of coronary atherosclerosis. Other researchers believe this particular HDL cholesterol is not protective. More research needs to be done, but the evidence seems to indicate *moderate* drinking does no damage to your heart.

THE STRESS RISK FACTOR

Few of us lead a life free of stress, but it's how we react—or overreact—to stress that makes the difference in our health.

The well-publicized Type-A personality is, in my opinion, not necessarily prone to coronary disease as is commonly assumed. A Type-A personality displays the following traits:

- Workaholic who works long hours with intensity.
- Overcommits himself and can't complete his work on time.
- Self-critical, easily angered, always impatient.
- Compulsive competitor who becomes upset if he doesn't win all the time.

I believe people who internalize their stress and anxiety are *more* at risk. They become angry and hostile, reacting with depression and despair over family or job stresses, with damaging results to their cardiovascular and cerebral-vascular systems. People like this are called *hot reactors,* a term introduced by Dr. Robert S. Eliot, a leading investigator of stress management. Hot reactors may be either Type-A or Type-B, but the Type-A hot reactor is at most risk for serious heart trouble. A comprehensive comparison between Type-A and Type-B personalities begins on page 143.

A hot reactor is a person who may or may not be hot-tempered but who is internally on a slow burn. His body's hormonal system overreacts to emotional stress, which affects his entire body because emotions communicate directly with the central nervous system, causing the brain to secrete hormones. These hormones are released whether emotions are positive or negative. With negative emotions, the body produces a considerably larger quantity of hormones.

Hormone production during times of stress is a biological throwback as a reaction to danger; stress hormones prepared the body to fight or flee. However, if you overreact now to a psychologically stressful situation at home or at the office, you overdose yourself with hormones because you aren't really fleeing or fighting.

Your central nervous system is activated by the secretion of *epinephrine* and *norepinephrine* substances (*adrenalin* is another of these hormones). Constant flow of excess hormones through the blood system to the heart and brain can overstimulate your nervous system. This may be detrimental to your health, and over time, it could result in heart damage.

Excess hormones cause your blood pressure to rise, sometimes alarmingly. Blood platelets collect more quickly, promoting blood clotting and thrombosis. (If you were actually wounded in battle this would be a good thing, but if you're sitting in your car in a traffic jam, it does you no good.) Excess hormones can result in more rapid progression of atherosclerosis. Over the years, small injuries to the heart muscle result in damage similar to that caused by an overt, painful heart attack.

In addition to this damage, norepinephrine secretion caused by anger and hostility can stimulate malignant rhythm disturbances in your heart in the form of ventricular fibrillation. This is the most common cause of sudden cardiac death. A father who dies unexpectedly from grief over his child's death may be a victim of ventricular fibrillation caused by an overwhelming discharge of hormones from the autonomic nervous system in reaction to his grief.

A "living study" of how stress affects health was done by Dr. Eliot at the Kennedy Space Center during the years NASA prepared to send an astronaut to the moon. The pace was frenzied; people were under intense stress. Records kept on workers at the space center revealed the divorce rate was 75%, alcohol consumption was the highest in the country, and the cardiac death rate among young men was 50% higher than an age-matched group of men not working at the center.

Conclusions by Dr. Eliot show the key factor in such a stressful situation is how stress was handled. A negative psychological reaction to stress on the job may cause detrimental health effects, such as high blood pressure, high pulse rate and irregularities in heart rhythm. In the most susceptible cases—hot-reactors—sudden cardiac death was the final, detrimental health effect.

SEX HORMONES MAY AFFECT HEART DISEASE

Women seem to be somewhat protected from heart disease until they reach menopause. The heart-attack rate in menstruating women is lower than in men of comparable age, but *after* menopause it rises rapidly to a rate close to that in men. This does not mean women below the age of menopause are immune to heart disease. They aren't, but their risk is considerably less than a man's.

Doctors believe the natural level of estrogen in a menstruating woman protects her from heart disease. It is unknown whether the estrogen reduces the effects of high blood pressure, smoking or high cholesterol, but it seems to play an important protective role. Artificial estrogen does not provide protection.

Recently a study based on Framingham data was reported at a conference of the American Heart Association. It showed post-menopausal women who take estrogen replacement therapy have a greater chance of developing heart disease or suffering a stroke than those who do not take estrogen. The subject is controversial.

Estrogen does not protect men from heart disease. In fact, when men who already have coronary insufficiency have taken estrogen experimentally, it made matters worse. Blood clots became more of a problem, and the rate of heart attacks was *not* reduced.

Although birth-control pills contain estrogen, they raise a woman's risk of heart disease considerably if she smokes and more subtly, but definitely, if she is over 40—even if she is a non-smoker. If a woman under 40 taking the pill does not smoke, she enjoys the same lower probabilities of heart disease as women who do not take the pill.

For the woman who smokes and takes the pill, chances of heart attack, stroke and phlebitis increase 8 to 10 times. I do not prescribe the pill for any woman who smokes.

Nor do I prescribe it for any woman who has high blood pressure or diabetes.

Other male and female hormones (testosterone and estradiol) are being studied by Dr. Gerald Phillips of Columbia University; he is attempting to determine if these hormones are involved in heart disease. One theory is that men whose hormones are subtly out of balance may be more susceptible to heart disease. This theory has generated considerable controversy, but no conclusions have been reached.

MULTIPLE RISK FACTORS COMPOUND YOUR RISK

If you have several risk factors for coronary disease, think long and hard about taking action to eliminate them. Statistics show people with multiple risk factors, such as hypertension, high cholesterol, obesity and inactivity, are at serious risk of developing a life-threatening condition.

When considering multiple risk factors, the risks are not simply added together. They are compounded. Evidence is too overwhelming to ignore; if you're at risk, act *now* before it's too late. Eliminate as many of the not-so-minor risk factors as you can because they add up to a big risk.

My risk-reducing nutrition plan and exercise program can help you gain control of your life. Follow these comprehensive programs, and you'll help improve your health and help lower your risks of heart disease and other debilitating diseases, such as cancer, diabetes and osteoporosis.

5.
LOWER YOUR RISK
OF HEART DISEASE

Don't wait until you suffer a heart attack before you face the facts about heart disease. Once heart disease is established, it's a difficult, frightening road back to good health. Prevention is an easier and surer path to follow. It takes many years of poor living habits to reach the point of heart disease, and it may take just as long to reverse the process.

You can lower your risk and protect yourself from heart disease by changing the factors that are dangerous to your heart's health. The factors that cause heart disease include cigarette smoking, hypertension, high serum-cholesterol levels, abnormal reaction to stress, obesity and diabetes. Other contributing factors, perhaps less statistically significant but still important, include excessive alcohol consumption, poor nutrition, overweight and physical inactivity.

Even if you have only one of these risk factors, you would be wise to eliminate it. If you have more than one, do something *now* because multiple risk factors compound your risk, and each worsens the effect of the other! Why wait to find out for certain your lifestyle is unhealthy? Why not follow the lead of scientific evidence and begin to reduce your risks now?

KICK THE SMOKING HABIT

If you smoke, all your efforts must be concentrated on stopping now! This isn't easy, but don't fool yourself. Your life may depend on kicking the habit.

49

In the United States, nearly 33% of all adults and 20% of all teenagers smoke cigarettes. Many would like to quit but can't because they're hooked. Whether you admit it or not, cigarette smoking is an addiction to nicotine, and it's a difficult habit to break.

Even if you're serious about quitting, odds are you won't be able to do it without professional help. The greatest successes in kicking the cigarette habit are achieved by people who join programs offered by the American Cancer Society, the American Heart Association or the National Lung Association. About 66% of the people who participate in these programs actually quit. But 1 year later, only 50% of the participants are still not smoking. These results are good when compared to the statistics of those who try to quit on their own. Only 20% have the habit still kicked 1 year after they "stopped."

A stop-smoking program helps you alter behavior associated with smoking. For instance, some smokers report they enjoy handling a cigarette at times of stress to have something to do with their hands. Other people enjoy a cup of coffee and a cigarette after a meal. Some people use cigarettes as a tranquilizer; others use them as stimulants. Still others are just in the habit of lighting up. In a stop-smoking program, you learn why you smoke and how to substitute healthier habits in place of smoking.

Behavior modification is important in breaking the cigarette habit, but it won't help you overcome your addiction to nicotine. Most people suffer nicotine-withdrawal symptoms. Some suffer badly; others hardly suffer at all. True nicotine addicts have a craving about every 20 minutes; if you quit smoking cold turkey, you're likely to suffer withdrawal symptoms for weeks.

Nicotine-withdrawal symptoms include headaches, lightheadedness, irritability, muscle cramps, food cravings, difficulty concentrating and extreme fatigue. But these don't last forever, and it is certainly preferable to suffer these for a while rather than have a heart attack.

A recently approved drug may help control smoking withdrawal symptoms. It is a nicotine-containing chewing gum, called *Nicorette,* that you can obtain with a prescription from your doctor. It's kind of like supplying methadone to a heroin addict. The gum allows you to concentrate on breaking all the behavior habits associated with smoking while you still get the "nicotine fix" your addicted body craves. Once you have modified your behavior, you begin to taper off using the chewing gum without suffering terribly from nicotine-withdrawal symptoms.

Studies show the gum is most effective when used in conjunction with a stop-smoking program. Six months after completing a stop-smoking program, 48% of the Nicorette users were no longer smoking, but only 20% of those who had used a placebo gum were no longer smoking. For those who were prescribed the gum, but who did not participate in a stop-smoking program, only 9% were not smoking 1 year later.

No matter how you finally quit smoking—even acupuncture and hypnosis work for some people—the greatest success rate is achieved by those who truly recognize the serious threat to their health that smoking poses.

The benefits gained by stopping smoking begin *immediately* after you quit, although you may not feel the difference for several weeks. Immediately after the effects of that last puff wear off, the carbon monoxide content of your blood drops, leaving more opportunity for oxygen to get into the red blood cells and circulate to your body and brain cells where oxygen is needed. The pathological effects and tissue damage caused by smoking slowly begin to reverse but take several months to be repaired.

It's never too late to stop smoking—and it's never too soon to stop either. Damage compounds with every cigarette you smoke. Giving up smoking is one of the most beneficial steps you can take to lower your chances of developing heart disease or arresting the disease once it begins.

BLOOD PRESSURE IS A KEY TO LONGEVITY

Studies of healthy elderly people show many have blood-pressure readings in the low end of the normal range. Some of these people may be genetically protected against developing arteriosclerosis and high blood pressure, or their healthy living habits may have prevented the condition. Whatever you do to keep your blood pressure under control will help you live longer and feel younger.

If you're overweight, that's the place to begin to lower your blood pressure. Reducing your weight to normal may bring mildly or moderately high blood pressure down to normal. Losing weight is not a simple matter for many of us—in the section that begins on page 204 you'll learn how to do it safely and effectively.

Don't try crash dieting because most of these diets can result in severe health problems and worsen high blood pressure and arteriosclerosis. Weight loss and blood-pressure control are best achieved by reducing calorie intake, reducing salt intake, getting adequate calcium and exercising regularly.

If your high blood pressure is related to stress, you may be able to lower it by modifying your personality. People who are hot-reactors or those with Type-A personalities can learn to control their emotions and lower their blood pressure through biofeedback, meditation and other relaxation techniques.

The answer lies in learning to harness your reaction to stress and avoiding unnecessary stress. Put life's priorities in order, and keep things in perspective. Don't become angry over things that are beyond your control, but try to solve your problems. Keep their importance in perspective so if you can't find a solution you don't overreact. Don't sweat the small things.

If you get overstressed, make a conscious effort to relax. Seek professional help if you need it; some people must *learn* to relax. Others need to discuss problems in group therapy, and some need to exercise regularly to dissipate stress hormones.

Drugs have a limited role in stress control but are often overused to smooth over problems. This may create greater stress because problems are not solved, and the patient gets no help in controlling his reacting type of personality. For drug use to be constructive, it should be combined with psychological counseling.

Tranquilizers, such as Valium and Librium, are frequently prescribed for stress. These work on the central nervous system, relieving anxiety and relaxing muscles. A class of compounds called *beta adrenergic blocking agents,* such as propranolol (Inderal), actually block the heart from reacting to norepinephrine and have a major role in protecting people with known heart conditions.

Some people use alcohol to control stress; they "need" it to relax. But alcohol can cause heart damage. Be careful not to depend on alcohol to cope with stress because you can't overcome unhappiness with alcohol.

Another important consideration in reducing stress as a risk factor is to weigh your goals. Think about how much you're pushing yourself to conform to society's pressures and pressures from your work and your family. Rethink your goals so you concentrate on what is really important to *you*—put the rest aside.

I firmly encourage exercise as a means of coping with stress, but don't confuse it with a solution. You can't "run away" from problems. Take the time to rethink and rediscover what you want to attain, where you want to go and how you plan to get there.

A recent national study, called the *MRFIT* (Multiple Risk Factor Intervention Trial) was sponsored by the National Heart and Blood Institute in Bethesda, Maryland. The results demonstrated the benefits and ease of controlling high blood pressure. Even lowering very mild elevations of blood pressure had beneficial effects on discouraging the development of cardiac and cerebral vascular disease as people aged.

YOU CAN LOWER YOUR CHOLESTEROL LEVEL

For many people, an elevated serum-cholesterol level is the overriding factor in development of heart disease. For others, it is a contributing factor along with other risk factors. Try to keep your cholesterol count as low as possible. It's vitally important to your health to limit cholesterol and saturated fat in your diet to maintain the lowest serum cholesterol and triglyceride levels possible.

Advertisers of cooking oil and margarine have made the words *cholesterol, unsaturated, saturated* and *polyunsaturated* part of our vocabulary. But what do these words mean and what do they have to do with heart disease?

Cholesterol is a fatty substance produced by your liver. Your body needs cholesterol to make hormones, other vital biochemicals and cell membranes. When present in your blood in excessive quantities, cholesterol is associated with vascular disease and arteriosclerosis. The higher the level of serum cholesterol, the greater your risk of heart disease. Most researchers agree the level of cholesterol in your blood is directly affected by your diet and the foods you commonly consume.

The most common, and highest, sources of cholesterol are:

- Egg yolk
- Butter, cheese, cream and whole-milk products
- Organ meats, such as liver, kidney and brain
- Beef, pork and lamb
- Sausage, bacon and processed luncheon meat
- Poultry skin (chicken, duck, turkey)

Many of the foods listed above are common in our diet. I'm not suggesting you never eat them, but the less you consume, the closer to ideal serum-cholesterol levels you can get. Limit egg yolks in *all* forms (from cake mixes to omelets) to three a week. Change from whole milk to skim milk. Use cheese made from skim goat milk. Eat less beef, and when you do eat it, cut all visible fat away *before* cooking. Avoid processed luncheon meat and sausage. Eat more chicken and fish, but don't fry them, and don't eat the skin.

Shellfish, such as scallops, shrimp and lobster, contain moderate levels of cholesterol—not the high levels they were once believed to have. About 30 large shrimp equal the cholesterol in one egg yolk!

Dietary fat comes in three forms:

- Saturated
- Monounsaturated
- Polyunsaturated

Fats of animal origin are saturated, and fats of vegetable origin are usually unsaturated. The difference between saturated and unsaturated is easy to understand. *Saturated* fat is solid at room temperature. *Unsaturated* fat is liquid at room temperature.

Oils that are "hydrogenated" (a process that makes them more solid at room temperature) means hydrogen is added to the fat molecule to make it more solid. This is done in making margarine and vegetable shortening; hydrogenation increases the saturated effect.

Saturated fats in your diet raise your serum-cholesterol levels, and unsaturated fats lower them. Polyunsaturated fats, which are the most unsaturated, were once believed to be the most effective cholesterol fighters, but recent research indicates monounsaturated fats may be more effective.

In a study of 20 patients, Dr. Scott Grundy of the University of Texas Health Science Center tested three diets—high saturated fat, high polyunsaturated fat and high monounsaturated fat. His research, published in the *Journal of Lipid Research,* showed monounsaturated fats lowered overall cholesterol levels the most. In addition, monounsaturated fats lowered the dangerous LDL-cholesterol fraction in relation to the protective HDL-cholesterol fraction, which provides further protection from heart disease.

A follow-up study by Dr. Grundy, published in the *New England Journal of Medicine,* adds further support to the importance of monounsaturated fats. Eleven middle-aged men and women followed three different diets. One diet was high in saturated fats, one was high in monounsaturated fats, and one was a low-fat diet. The monounsaturated diet lowered cholesterol levels by 13%, while the low-fat diet lowered cholesterol levels by only 8%. In addition, the monounsaturated fats increased the proportion of protective HDL cholesterol.

Saturated fat is almost always found in the same foods that contain high levels of cholesterol, except shellfish, which have very little fat. The oils and fats in plants (vegetables, fruits, nuts and grains) are usually unsaturated, except for palm oil and coconut oil, which are saturated and should be avoided. Read labels on packaged foods because they frequently contain palm or coconut oils. Avoid prepared foods with these fats. The chart below shows the fats found in many foods we eat.

Many people create their own problems with cholesterol by eating too many fatty foods full of saturated fat and cholesterol. Research indicates that when the body is frequently supplied with saturated fat, the liver's cholesterol production increases. On the other hand, reliable experiments show that substituting unsaturated for saturated dietary fats either reduces the rate of cholesterol production or promotes excretion of the cholesterol produced.

To lower your serum-cholesterol level, your total daily intake of ready-made cholesterol should be limited to about 300mg. One egg yolk contains about 250mg of

Fats Ranked in Order of Saturation

	Iodine #	Fats
	10	Coconut—9
	20	Ice cream—20
		Cheese—American, Cheddar, blue, Camembert—20
		Milk, whole—23
	30	Butter—33
SATURATED		Chocolate—37
FAT	40	Lamb—40
	50	Beef—57
		Shortening, animal—59
	60	Lard—64
		Bacon—67
	70	Shortening, vegetable—70
	80	Eggs—84
		Olive oil—84
		Turkey—84
MONOUNSATURATED	90	Chicken—92
FAT	100	Peanut butter—100
		Peanut oil—100
	110	Tuna—110
	120	Halibut (liver)—120
		Corn oil—127
		Wheat germ—129
	130	Soy bean oil—133
POLYUNSATURATED		Sunflower oil—134
FAT	140	Safflower oil—146
	150	Salmon (body)—151
	160	English walnut oil—162
	170	Codfish (liver)—178

cholesterol, so restrict eggs. I usually allow my patients a total of three or four eggs a week.

Eat only small quantities of foods high in saturated fats and cholesterol. Choose margarine over butter, and use margarines that are high in polyunsaturates (those usually made from corn or safflower oil). Soft-tub margarines made from corn, sunflower or safflower oils have the least hydrogenation and are the best to use.

Choose polyunsaturated and monounsaturated cooking and salad oils. Olive oil is monounsaturated and should be used often in salad dressings and cooking. Foods to avoid include packaged baked goods—cakes, pies, crackers and cookies. These often contain animal fat (lard).

Even products with labels that boast they are made from vegetable shortening may not be healthy for your heart. Fine print may reveal coconut and palm oils, which you want to avoid. Dairy substitutes, such as whipped toppings and coffee creamers, also contain coconut and palm oils.

You can't eat as much unsaturated fat as you want. Some research indicates diets high in unsaturated fat, polyunsaturated fat in particular, can cause certain kinds of cancer.

I usually recommend to my patients that their diet consist of 1/3 saturated fat, 1/3 monounsaturated fat and 1/3 polyunsaturated fat. Total fat consumption in your daily diet should be no more than 20% of the calories you consume. If you consume 2,000 calories a day, you should be eating 400 calories (45 grams) of fat. This is discussed in the section that explains the risk-reducing nutrition plan that begins on page 186.

Recent research has shown two polyunsaturated fats, called *omega-3 fatty acids*, are found in fatty cold-water fish. These fats dramatically lower serum-cholesterol levels and reduce clotting tendencies, which can help protect you from heart disease.

Scientists became curious about these fats because Eskimos in Alaska and Greenland eat more fat than anyone else in the world, but they rarely have heart attacks. Analyses of their diets showed the dietary fat comes from cold-water fish.

Research studies from Harvard University, the Oregon Health Sciences University and the University of Leiden in the Netherlands indicate the consumption of omega-3 fats, specifically eicosapentanoic acid (EPA) and docosahexaenoic acid (DHA), reduces the stickiness and clotting tendency of the blood platelets. Clotting can form dangerous artery-clogging thromboses and cause heart attack and stroke. When the clotting tendency is reduced, arterial walls become more resistant to the buildup of cholesterol placques. Omega-3 fats also lower serum levels of triglycerides and very-low-density cholesterol and reduce production of cholesterol-carrying proteins in the liver.

Fish that contain these protective fats include salmon, mackeral, bluefish, tuna, swordfish, sardines, mullet, herring, sablefish, trout, shad, butterfish and pompano. Shellfish, which was once forbidden for those on a low-cholesterol diet, contain some protective omega-3 fatty acids. The amount of cholesterol shellfish contain has recently been shown to be less than was originally believed, so you can safely eat them in moderation.

Include the fatty cold-water fish regularly in your diet—2 or 3 times a week is recommended. Clams, mussels, oysters and scallops, which are very low in cholesterol, may be eaten freely.

How you cook your fish is important; steam or poach it. It's permissible to pan-fry or broil fish with small amounts of fat. Deep frying or serving fish in creamy sauces counteracts the benefits of this cholesterol-lowering seafood!

Smoked and pickled fish contain large amounts of salt and possibly cancer-causing chemicals. Avoid them, and choose fish prepared in more nutritious ways. Water-packed tuna is a good choice as long as you don't need to avoid salt, but low-salt brands are available.

If you prefer steak to fish, you may feel it's a good idea to take fish oil in capsule form and keep on eating your beef. Some fish-oil capsules, such as maxEPA, are sold in health-food stores or through the mail, but I don't recommend them.

Don't be fooled into thinking you can continue to eat your normal fatty diet of steak, roast beef, butter and whipped cream, then protect yourself by swallowing a few fish-oil capsules. It doesn't work that way. The benefit comes from *removing* bad fats from your diet and substituting good ones. Furthermore, no one can tell you what is a safe dosage of fish oil. It's possible to ingest toxic amounts of vitamin A and vitamin D from taking these capsules. It's healthier and less expensive to eat fish!

Sometimes changing dietary habits isn't enough. Some people have overt, inherited problems involving metabolism of fats and sugar. They overproduce cholesterol, fail to transport it to the right destination or cannot adequately clear it from their arteries. Dietary changes in these people do not offer much help. In the case of someone with truly abnormal blood-lipid levels, a doctor should prescribe cholesterol-lowering drugs and a strict low-fat diet. But for all others, the risk-reducing nutrition plan and risk-reducing exercise plan provide the keys to help protect the heart's arteries.

EXERCISE MAY SAVE YOUR HEART

Aerobic exercise is crucial to keeping your heart in good condition. Every research study that compares inactive with active people shows inactive individuals have higher heart-attack rates than those who are active.

Physically active people who get aerobic exercise have fewer heart attacks and lower death rates from heart disease. Active people are more likely to live longer, healthier and more-productive lives.

Fitness is not a guaranteed immunity from heart disease. The death of Jim Fixx, the author of *Running* and an early popularizer of jogging, demonstrated this fact. Fixx was burdened with a serious family history of early heart disease and was once overweight and a smoker. He was known to have eaten a high-fat diet.

By becoming physically fit, Fixx probably lengthened his life considerably, but his fitness could not compensate totally for his genetic tendencies. If he had not refused to undergo an exercise stress test, which would have revealed the condition of his heart, he might be alive today. Proper diagnosis and treatment could have protected him further.

Many of us lead sedentary lives, so getting enough exercise and finding the time to include exercise in a daily routine can be a problem. For most the question is, "What is the minimum amount of exercise I can do and still protect my cardiovascular system?" Do you really need to jog 10 miles, 5 times a week? Or can you play a relaxed game of tennis 3 times a week? The answer varies according to your present health.

A young man, somewhat overweight, trying to break a cigarette habit and trying to improve the level of his blood lipoprotein level, would have to exercise more vigorously and more often than a person of the same age who had no risk factors. It would not be a waste of time for the first man to exercise in a more-relaxed way because some benefit is achieved simply by not being sedentary. But for him, the most benefit would come from fairly strenuous exercise.

You can achieve cardiac fitness by *aerobically* working the large-muscle groups in your legs, thighs and arms. That means running, swimming, dancing or moving in any way that increases your pulse and requires deep breathing, causing you to take in more oxygen. To be effective, aerobic exercise must increase your heart rate for an extended period of time—at least 10 to 15 minutes. If your body is not in good physical shape, begin your exercise program gradually.

YOU CAN HAVE A DRINK NOW AND THEN

Moderate amounts of alcohol may protect you from heart disease, but as previously discussed, drinking more than moderately gradually damages your cardiovascular system. Heavy drinking can do severe damage.

Moderate alcohol consumption means you don't exceed an average of 3 ounces of hard liquor, two 5-ounce glasses of wine or two 12-ounce glasses of beer 5 days a week. That may be a lot of alcohol or a drop in the bucket compared to how much you usually drink.

If you drink more than moderately, cut down. Instead of a mixed drink, have club soda and lime. Switch to light beer if you can't reduce the number of beers you drink. Learn to sip and savor your wine. If you can't do this on your own, you have a drinking problem and should seek professional help.

Recent studies show people who have high HDL-cholesterol levels, which protect against heart disease, are often moderate drinkers. Moderate drinkers are less likely to get heart disease than people who do not drink at all or people who drink a great deal. This fact has led people to conclude that alcohol is safe for the heart, but this idea must be tempered with the guidelines of moderation. I don't advise a non-drinker to begin drinking to protect his heart. But if you enjoy alcohol within moderate limits, statistics are in your favor for achieving a better level of HDL cholesterol. This level seems protective against future coronary heart disease.

EFFECTS OF ASPIRIN AND OTHER SUBSTANCES

Perhaps you've heard that an aspirin a day protects your heart. Some research suggests this may be true, but the evidence is not yet conclusive. Aspirin and several other related drugs interfere with the blood-clotting mechanisms of blood platelets. Platelets are essential to clogging up a wounded blood vessel but may clog excessively in the heart's arteries *after* there has been some disruption of the very smooth coronary-artery walls.

Most men over 40 probably have some arteriosclerosis; reducing the platelets' tendency to clot may prevent further buildup of fatty debris and blood clots in their arteries. This may reduce the likelihood of heart attack.

Aspirin would be a simple, inexpensive preventive for heart disease, but too much aspirin knocks out the body's mechanism for preventing heart disease. We don't know how much aspirin is "the right amount." One study indicated 20mg (one aspirin is 325mg) was the proper amount. Another found 40mg sufficient, and another recommended one aspirin every other day. The right amount has not been determined, so don't self-prescribe an aspirin a day for heart disease.

Some people are sensitive to aspirin—their stomachs bleed profusely from taking aspirin regularly. They may not know it until they've bled a large amount. Aspirin can also cause ringing in the ears; long-term use may result in permanent ear damage.

In special situations supervised by your doctor, aspirin therapy may be advisable. But don't take aspirin unsupervised by your doctor as a protection against heart attacks; you might cause damage to your body. Be patient. The answer will come from carefully done studies within the next few years. If you already have heart disease, your doctor must decide if it is appropriate for you to take aspirin now.

Stimulants, if used with regularity, can cause hypertension. Benzedrine, cocaine, amphetamine, over-the-counter diet aids, and cold remedies and decongestants that contain stimulants may raise blood pressure. Read labels for warnings.

If you have elevated blood pressure, certain drugs can make it significantly abnormal, so avoid taking anything indiscriminately until you have consulted with your doctor. If you have early asymptomatic heart disease, these drugs might hasten development of significantly severe disease.

LOSE WEIGHT NOW

Obesity is an added burden on the heart. Coupled with high blood pressure, overweight more than doubles the increased risk of congestive heart failure. Even in people who do not have high blood pressure or high cholesterol, the incidence of heart disease is greater if they are obese than if they are of normal weight.

Obese people have a discouraging success rate when it comes to losing weight. But if you're overweight, you must diet safely to lose weight. My permanent weight-loss diet plan works best for motivated people who are overweight but not dangerously obese.

If you are truly obese and have been unsuccessful in losing weight and keeping it off, seek professional help before it is too late. Often a psychotherapist is the key to success in teaching an obese person how to control his lifestyle and eating habits.

YOU CAN MAKE UP FOR PAST SINS

If you have smoked, been physically lazy and eaten poorly, is it worth your while to change? The answer is a definite *yes!* Statistics of men who stopped smoking *after* suffering a heart attack, compared to a similar group of men who did not stop smoking, show those who stopped lived longer and were less likely to have a second heart attack.

If you stop smoking before you have a heart attack, it will do you even more good. Anyone who stops smoking *now* is less likely to develop heart disease than his counterpart who continues smoking. The earlier in life you stop smoking, the greater the benefit. All statistics, whether they relate to cancer or heart disease, indicate beneficial effects begin immediately following cessation of smoking.

The same goes for people who begin to exercise (properly and with medical clearance) after being sedentary. Benefits to the heart—lower blood pressure, lower weight, lower cholesterol, higher oxygen consumption, improved fitness levels—are a healthy consequence of regular vigorous exercise, no matter when you begin.

If you have eaten too much fat and cholesterol in the past, you *can* reverse the damage. Experimental evidence indicates cholesterol is constantly being deposited on and removed from artery walls. Once put there, it is not necessarily a permanent fixture. You can slowly reverse the damage as long as your habits change adequately and permanently!

If you are at risk of heart disease, the news is good. You can take steps now to help reduce your risks. Change your diet, lower your blood pressure, lose weight, stop smoking, drink moderately and start exercising!

6.

THE RISK FACTORS OF STROKE

TAKE THIS TEST TO MEASURE YOUR
STROKE RISK

This test measures your risk of suffering a stroke. Circle the score for each characteristic that applies to you. Total the score, then check your risk category on page 63.

Personal

Choose any that apply.

+1   You are male

+2   You are black

+5   You take birth-control pills, smoke cigarettes and are under 40

+8   You take birth-control pills, smoke cigarettes and are over 40

+10   You take birth-control pills and smoke cigarettes

+12   You take birth control pills, smoke cigarettes, have high blood pressure and are black

+2   You are overweight by 20%

+4   You are overweight by 30%

+4   You are diabetic

+1   You do not engage in regular, vigorous exercise

Blood Pressure

Choose any that apply.

Your blood pressure is:

0	Below 120/75
+1	120/75 to 140/85
+2	140/85 to 150/90
+6	150/90 to 175/100
+10	175/100 to 190/110
+12	Over 190/110
+2	Your blood pressure is presently normal but is controlled by medication
+3	Elevated blood pressure first noted at about 180/110 and has not been controlled by medication or other means below 150/90
+6	Elevated blood pressure first noted at 210/120 and has not been controlled by medication or other means below 160/100
+5	Elevated blood pressure first noted before age 35 and not effectively kept below 140/95 since detection

Diet

Choose any that apply.

+1	You eat fatty cuts of steak, hamburger, pork and/or lamb 3 or more times a week
+1	You eat fatty processed meats, such as bologna, sausage or ham, 2 or more times a week
+1	You eat generous amounts of butter or margarine
+1	You eat fried foods several times a week
+1	You eat rich desserts or ice cream several times a week
+1	You drink more than 2 glasses of whole milk a day
+1	You eat cheese (except low-fat cottage cheese) several times a week
+1	You salt food during cooking but not at the table
+2	You taste food first but often add salt
+3	You salt food at the table before tasting it
+5	You salt food at the table and have blood pressure over 120/75
+2	You frequently eat salty foods, such as pickles, chips or nuts, or you frequently eat prepared or restaurant foods

Family History

Choose any that apply.

+6   Mother or father suffered a stroke before age 45

+4   Mother or father suffered a stroke between age 45 and 55

+2   Mother or father suffered a stroke between age 55 and 65

+4   Both parents suffered a stroke before age 65

Smoking

Choose one.

0   You never smoked, or quit over 5 years ago

+1   You quit smoking 1 to 5 years ago

+2   You quit smoking during the past year

+2   You smoke 1/2 to 1 pack of cigarettes a day

+3   You smoke 1 to 2 packs of cigarettes a day

+5   You smoke more than 2 packs of cigarettes a day

+1   You began smoking within the last year

+2   You now smoke or quit within the last year and began smoking within the last 5 years

+3   You now smoke or quit within the last year and began smoking 5 to 10 years ago

+5   You now smoke or quit within the last year and began smoking more than 20 years ago as an adult

+8   You now smoke or quit within the last year and began smoking more than 20 years ago as a teenager

Stress

Choose any that apply.

+3   As the primary breadwinner of the family, you are very concerned you may not achieve the level of family income you desire within the next 5 years

+3   You are under age 65 and feel the pressure of constant work overload

+3   You are emotionally volatile, experience uncontrollable temper and feel angry

+3   You frequently feel tense and suppress your anger

+3   You are a housewife and mother and work long hours without feeling emotional support or satisfaction from your family

INTERPRETING YOUR SCORE

To determine your score, add all scores from the categories. Check your total score below to see if your health and your life are at risk. You may be referred to the risk-reducing nutrition plan, page 186, or the risk-reducing exercise plan, page 226.

0 to 7   **Low Risk**—You are at low risk of suffering a stroke. Your family history and lifestyle offer you the greatest protection.

8 to 19   **Moderate Risk**—You are at moderate risk of suffering a stroke. If your family history puts you at risk, follow the risk-reducing nutrition plan, stop smoking and get regular exercise to help lower your risk.

20 to 34   **High Risk**—You are at high risk of suffering a stroke. Be aware of any warning signs, such as dizziness, slurred speech or numbness on one side of your body. See a doctor *immediately* if any of these symptoms occur. You can help lower your risks by controlling elevated blood pressure and having it checked regularly. Follow the risk-reducing nutrition and exercise plans, and stop smoking.

35+   **Very High Risk**—You are at very high risk of suffering a stroke. Be aware of any warning signs, such as dizziness, slurred speech or numbness on one side of your body. See a doctor *immediately* if any of these symptoms occur. Though there's nothing you can do about an unfavorable family history, you can help lower risks by controlling elevated blood pressure and having it checked regularly. Follow the risk-reducing nutrition plan and the risk-reducing exercise plan, and stop smoking.

The Risk Factors of Stroke

Every year, 400,000 people in the United States suffer a stroke; 160,000 of them die soon after the stroke. The other 240,000 recover to lead limited, restricted lives. Stroke is our third leading killer, after heart disease and cancer, but it is often preventable. You don't *have* to be among its victims if you take steps now to help lower your risk.

A stroke is brain damage that results from vascular disease caused by a *brain hemorrhage* or a blockage or blood clot in a blood vessel, called a *thrombosis*. The clot forms in a vein or elsewhere and moves through the bloodstream, lodging in the brain. In either case, the disease is a form of hardening of the arteries.

A remarkable arrangement of vessels supplies your brain with blood. The main vessels lead directly from the heart; they are the *carotid arteries,* one on each side of the throat, and the *vertebral (basilar) arteries,* going up the back of the neck through the muscles. These vessels branch out in the brain. Blood drains back to the heart through the *jugular veins.*

Certain parts of the carotid and vertebral arteries appear to be vulnerable to hemorrhage because most hemorrhages occur in the same locations. This suggests turbulence and pressure within the arteries may weaken the arterial wall. If your blood pressure is higher than normal, blood coursing through these arteries is under higher pressure. This causes constant stress and strain on the arterial walls, especially on vulnerable spots, which may result in a stroke caused by cerebral hemorrhage.

Only a small percentage of people with hypertension (high blood pressure) suffer strokes. The brain is well-protected and can tolerate great variations in blood pressure without ill-effect. Only after long periods of abnormally high pressure will some people experience cerebral hemorrhage.

Thrombosis may also occur when carotid and vertebral arteries become clogged with cholesterol deposits. Although these arteries are outside the brain, they supply the blood the brain requires. If these arteries become clogged, the brain is deprived of blood, and stroke and brain damage can result.

Clogging of these arteries results from the same conditions that cause heart disease—a high-fat diet, overweight, smoking, high blood pressure, lack of exercise. Women who take birth-control pills, who also have high blood pressure or who smoke cigarettes, have an increased risk of stroke due to migrating blood clots. Birth-control pills should be discontinued if high blood pressure develops. In addition, women who take estrogen replacement have a greater risk of stroke than similar women who do not take estrogen.

The most serious risk factor for stroke is hypertension. Obesity, diabetes and pre-existing heart disease are also important risk factors of stroke. If there is a history of stroke in your family, you are at greater risk. A family history of stroke suggests the possibility you might have a genetic predilection for a weakness of the blood vessels;

you must make every effort you possibly can to protect your vascular system.

You can reduce your risk of stroke by the same methods used for preventing heart disease. Your aim is to reduce hardening of the arteries and lower your blood pressure. To do this, stop smoking, follow a low-fat diet, stay physically active and control your reactions to stress. Although statistics related to the cause of stroke, and thus its prevention, are not as significant as those pertaining to heart disease, it is evident *any* measure taken to reduce vascular atherosclerosis reduces your risk of stroke.

THE HYPERTENSION RISK FACTOR

Hypertension is the outstanding risk factor for development of stroke. The incidence of hypertension is similar between the sexes; women experience blood-pressure elevation and its complications as often as men. Women using birth-control pills are at risk of hypertension and stroke as a side effect of the pill; they should be aware of this potential complication. The same warning applies to post-menopausal women taking estrogen-replacement medication.

There are two types of high blood pressure—*secondary hypertension* and *primary (essential) hypertension.* Secondary hypertension is caused by disease elsewhere in the body, such as kidney disease or a tumor in the adrenal gland or pituitary gland. High blood pressure can also be caused by drugs or medication, but the high blood pressure is a secondary reaction to another condition. Secondary hypertension can often be controlled by treating the cause.

Primary hypertension is most common, but its cause is unknown. It is an illness and is not caused by another treatable condition. Many factors are associated with primary hypertension, and this is where we will focus our attention.

Being overweight, ingesting too much sodium, getting too little calcium, over-reacting to stress, consuming too much alcohol and having a family history of primary hypertension are all risk factors for development of primary hypertension. Except for family history, these risk factors are due to your lifestyle, but who knows if your family's history of hypertension isn't due to unhealthy lifestyle habits you learned? It's up to you to change your lifestyle.

As we age, our arterial system begins to become a bit more rigid and narrowed. There is a tendency for blood pressure to rise. When this happens, a condition of systolic hypertension develops. Doctors once regarded this as normal and of no concern. We now know elevated systolic blood pressure does constitute a risk of heart disease and stroke and should not be ignored. We also know elderly people with excellent cardiovascular health do not necessarily experience elevated systolic blood pressure. It *is* an avoidable part of aging.

YOU CAN LOWER BLOOD PRESSURE NATURALLY

It is possible, and desirable, to lower blood pressure by natural means rather than by resorting to drugs. You may be able to do this by following a low-salt, high-calcium diet, losing weight if necessary, controlling your reaction to stress and getting adequate exercise. When these methods fail, it becomes necessary to use medication to lower blood pressure.

Losing weight may also help lower blood pressure—it can often completely control hypertension in overweight people. If you have high blood pressure and are overweight, take off some pounds! The benefits of weight loss apply to so many areas of your health that you really have no excuse.

In the overweight person with high blood pressure, weight should be lost by calorie reduction, exercise *and* sodium restriction. Exercise according to your doctor's advice and under his supervision. When combined, this program creates benefits beyond lowering blood pressure. Weight loss must *not* be accomplished by fad or gimmick diets because these can cause further ill-health and raise blood pressure even higher. You must lose weight with the serious intent of making long-term changes in your dietary habits. You need to reduce calories and eat a nourishing, well-balanced diet. I tell you how to lose weight permanently, without risk, in the section that begins on page 204.

We consume too much sodium in salty foods and food additives, such as MSG (monosodium glutamate). Many researchers believe a high-sodium diet causes elevated blood pressure in susceptible people. Many of our favorite snack foods are salty; fast foods and convenience foods are loaded with excess sodium, and we are often careless with the salt shaker! Reducing sodium consumption has been advocated for everyone! If followed, this might lower blood-pressure readings for many people.

Some people can consume as much sodium as they like—up to 15 grams a day (2 grams of sodium is recommended)—and not develop high blood pressure. On the other hand, some people can eat the same amount and feel no different but have hypertension related only to excessive sodium intake.

At this time, there is no way to predict who is susceptible to sodium-induced high blood pressure and who is not. It seems prudent for everyone to lower sodium intake and have blood pressure checked regularly.

Your body requires sodium to function, but it's almost impossible to eat an ordinary diet *without* consuming adequate amounts of sodium. And that applies to athletes and people who do heavy physical work and perspire profusely! Your body has a unique capacity to save all the sodium it needs.

If you make a conscious effort to limit sodium, the health benefits are very real. If you don't use salt at the table and if you avoid frequent consumption of high-sodium foods, you are practicing preventive medicine.

Some people are addicted to salt, but it is an addiction that can be broken. If you gradually cut down the amount of salt you add to your food, when cooking and at the table, you won't notice the difference. The taste you have for salt is an acquired taste; after you break the habit, food that once tasted good to you will taste overly salty!

If your doctor puts you on a low-sodium diet, you must take further steps than those described above to reduce your sodium intake. Avoid *all* salty, prepared meats, such as luncheon meat and ham. Replace processed, packaged and canned foods with low-sodium brands, and restrict cheese and dairy products.

Physical and psychological stress can also cause an elevation in blood pressure. This is not necessarily a cause of hypertension but is a natural reaction to the hormones your body releases when you react to fear or anger. When you overreact to everyday stress with undue anger, resentment and worry, you are overloading your body with stress hormones. Your chances of chronic blood-pressure elevation are significant.

A person who overreacts to stress is called a hot-reactor and is often described as likely to "blow a gasket." A hot-reactor may suffer from a stroke or heart attack during a fit of temper because of the harmful effects of elevated blood pressure.

Often people with this type of personality resort to alcohol to relax. We probably all know someone who often has a drink or two to help him relax after a demanding day of work. Ironically, alcohol is a contributor to elevated blood pressure when used frequently and when used under stress. So avoid alcohol if you are under stress.

Another approach to lowering elevated blood pressure by natural means is to incorporate regular physical activity into your daily routine. Regular exercise causes a substantial reduction of blood pressure independent of any anti-hypertensive medication you might take.

Exercise can also influence blood pressure. In one study, hypertensives who started with blood pressures about 150/100 and exercised regularly reduced their average blood pressure to 135/85 with exercise alone.

Many sedentary people's muscles are virtually unused and contain beds of narrowed or closed-off capillaries, which cause elevated blood pressure. These capillaries can be opened up permanently through regular exercise, lowering the vascular resistance to blood flow and enabling the heart to push blood more easily to the peripheries of the body.

Exercise also benefits the circulation by reducing the effect of stress hormones. When you're under stress, your system produces more adrenalinlike hormones, which cause your arteries to clamp down and impede circulation, thus raising blood pressure. Aerobic exercise uses up these hormones before they can do you any harm.

HYPERTENSION CAN BE TREATED WITH MEDICATION

If natural means of lowering blood pressure don't work adequately, then it's essential for you, if you have consistently elevated blood-pressure readings above

140/90, to take anti-hypertensive medication under your doctor's supervision. A wide variety of medicinal approaches to hypertension control is now available; your doctor can choose the best method for you.

The medications used most often are diurectics, which reduce fluid volume and permit the excretion of excess sodium and water from the body. Potassium and calcium are also lost, along with harmful sodium, and should be replaced with mineral supplements or through a diet rich in potassium and calcium. The risk-reducing nutrition plan, page 186, is high in potassium and calcium.

Some doctors now use beta-blocker drugs as the first line of defense in controlling hypertension. These remarkable drugs offer many health benefits—they lower blood pressure, lower oxygen demand, slow the pulse and reduce tension-migraine headaches—all with a minimum of unpleasant side effects. Several different beta-blockers are presently available, and each is capable of lowering blood pressure to normal. Your doctor will choose the best one for you; if you can't tolerate one, another will probably work for you. Both diuretics and beta-blocker drugs used for long periods may have adverse effects on your lipid patterns, raising your serum-cholesterol level. Your doctor will keep a close watch on your blood-cholesterol level.

A newer class of compounds, called *calcium antagonists,* are also being used to control hypertension. There are dozens of other preparations available; your physician will tailor a prescription to your requirements. He will take into account the degree of your hypertension and any other complicating factors.

Another drug being studied in the prevention of stroke is aspirin. Aspirin prevents blood clots, so it may be beneficial in stroke prevention, but it should not be self-prescribed because it can cause serious internal bleeding. Aspirin use in vascular-disease prevention is still experimental and should be used *only* under medical supervision!

Many people at risk of stroke experience warning signs. If you experience a weakness on one side of your body or face, have fleeting episodes of speech impairment, visual disturbances, headache, dizziness, drowsiness and even personality changes, see your doctor immediately! Medical intervention may prevent a stroke and save your life.

If you are at risk of stroke, protect yourself by taking steps now to lower your blood pressure. Under your doctor's supervision, follow a low-sodium, low-fat diet, lose weight if necessary and begin an exercise program. The risk-reducing nutrition plan and the risk-reducing exercise plan, page 226, will help you lower your risk of stroke. The time to start is *now!*

7.

THE MAJOR RISK FACTORS OF CANCER

TAKE THIS TEST TO MEASURE YOUR
OVERALL CANCER RISKS

The tests in this section evaluate your risks of developing various forms of cancer. Take each test to evaluate your risk of a particular form of cancer.

This test measures your overall chance of having cancer. Circle the score for each characteristic that applies to you. Total the score, then check your risk category on page 72.

Family History

Choose any that apply.

+2   One parent, aunt, uncle, grandparent or sibling with cancer
+15 More than one close relative with cancer
+10 One or more close relative with cancer, and *you* smoke cigarettes, cigars or a pipe
+15 One or more close relatives with cancer, and *you* smoke cigarettes, cigars or a pipe, *and* drink more than one or two 5-ounce glasses of wine or 12-ounce glasses of beer or 3 ounces of hard liquor a day, more than 5 days a week
+1   You drink more than two cups of caffeinated or decaffeinated coffee a day *and* have a close relative who had pancreatic cancer

69

Smoking

Choose any that apply.

+1 Smoke less than 1 pack of cigarettes a day

+5 Smoke 1 pack of cigarettes a day

+8 Smoke 2 or more packs of cigarettes a day

+10 Smoke 1 or more packs of cigarettes a day and drink two or three 5-ounce glasses of wine or 12-ounce glasses of beer or 3 ounces of hard liquor a day, 5 or more days a week

+2 Smoke cigars or a pipe

+4 Smoke cigars or a pipe and drink two or three 5-ounce glasses of wine or 12-ounce glasses of beer or 3 ounces of hard liquor a day, 5 or more days a week

+2 Live *or* work with smokers

+3 Live *and* work with smokers

+1 Live *or* work in heavily air-polluted area

+2 Live *and* work in heavily air-polluted area

Personal

Choose any that apply.

+8 Sunburn easily and have had one or more severe sunburns with peeling, blistered skin

+5 Do not tan easily and are exposed to strong sun only occasionally, such as during vacations or on weekends

+3 Overweight by 20%

+5 Overweight by 25% or more

+1 Have been overweight most of your life

+2 Known exposure to pesticides, toxic wastes or asbestos in air, water or soil

+3 Have had many diagnostic X-rays in your life, especially when young

+4 Drink more than three 5-ounce glasses of wine or 12-ounce glasses of beer or 3 ounces of hard liquor a day, more than 5 days a week

+2 Lead a sedentary life without any regular, vigorous exercise

+1 Often feel lonely or isolated from other people

+1 Have no close friends or loved ones

+1 Feel depressed or overwhelmed much of the time

Diet

Choose any that apply.

−5   Do not eat meat

+1   Eat steak, hamburger, pork and/or lamb 3 times a week

+2   Eat steak, hamburger, pork and/or lamb 5 times a week

+3   Eat steak, hamburger, pork and/or lamb more than 5 times a week

+2   Eat processed meats, such as bologna, sausage or ham, twice a week

+3   Eat processed meats, such as bologna, sausage or ham, 3 to 5 times a week

+4   Eat processed meats, such as bologna, sausage or ham, more than 5 times a week

+2   Eat smoked or charcoal-grilled foods more than once a week

+1   Eat generous amounts of butter or margarine

+1   Eat fried foods several times a week

+2   Eat fried foods almost every day

+1   Eat rich desserts or ice cream several times a week

+2   Eat rich desserts or ice cream almost every day

+1   Drink at least 1 to 2 glasses of *whole* milk, or the equivalent, each day

+1   Eat cheese (except low-fat cottage cheese) several times a week

+2   Eat cheese (except low-fat cottage cheese) almost every day

+2   Eat empty-calorie foods or processed food several times a week

+4   Eat empty-calorie foods or processed food almost every day

+2   Eat less than 2 slices of whole-grain bread a day

+3   Eat high-fiber cereal less than 3 times a week

+3   Eat less than 3 servings of fruits or vegetables a day

+3   Do not drink citrus juice or eat a citrus fruit every day

+3   Eat broccoli, cabbage, cauliflower or Brussels sprouts less than 3 times a week

---
INTERPRETING YOUR SCORE

To determine your score, add all scores from the categories. Check your total score below to see if your health and your life are at risk. You may be referred to the risk-reducing nutrition plan, page 186, or the risk-reducing exercise plan, page 226.

0 to 14   **Low Risk**—Your risk of cancer is low because you eat a proper diet, exercise and live a healthier lifestyle.

15 to 25   **Moderate Risk**—You have a moderate risk of developing cancer. To help lower your risk, follow the risk-reducing nutrition plan, stop smoking and begin an exercise program *now*.

26 to 35   **High Risk**—Your lifestyle is conspiring against you to raise your risk of cancer. Stop smoking now! Follow the risk-reducing nutrition plan and the risk-reducing exercise plan, and you may significantly lower your risk.

36+   **Very High Risk**—Your family history and your unhealthy lifestyle are putting you at very high risk of cancer. If you change your ways now, stop smoking and begin the risk-reducing nutrition plan and risk-reducing exercise plan, you can help lower your risk considerably.

TAKE THIS TEST TO MEASURE YOUR COLON-CANCER RISK

This test measures your risk of developing cancer of the colon (large bowel). Circle the score for each characteristic that applies to you. Total the score, then check your risk category on page 74.

Family History

Choose any that apply.

   +3   One or more close relative with colon cancer or colon polyps, and you *do not* have colon polyps

   +5   One or more close relative with colon cancer or colon polyps, and you have colon polyps

Diet

Choose any that apply.

+2   Eat beef almost every day

+3   Eat whole-milk dairy products, such as cheese, butter, cream cheese, ice cream or whole milk, about 3 times a week

+5   Eat whole-milk dairy products, such as cheese, butter, cream cheese, ice cream or whole milk, every day or almost every day

+3   Eat fried or butter-sauce foods several times or more a week

+5   Eat fried or butter-sauce foods every day

+3   Eat pastries or rich desserts several times a week

+5   Eat pastries or rich desserts every day

+4   Eat high-fat, empty-calorie foods, such as chips, dips and French fries, several times a week

+3   Eat white bread rather than whole-grain bread

−3   Eat a high-fiber cereal almost every day

−3   Eat more than 3 servings of fruits or vegetables every day

−3   Eat broccoli, cauliflower, cabbage or Brussels sprouts several times a week

Personal

Choose any that apply.

+3   You have a history of ulcerative colitis

+2   You are frequently constipated

+3   You have small, loose or ribbonlike stools

+2   You are under considerable stress at work or home and are frequently constipatéd or have diarrhea

−1   You exercise vigorously for 30 minutes or more 5 or more days a week.

+3   You are male and overweight by 20%

+1   You are overweight and have been all or most of your adult life

---
INTERPRETING YOUR SCORE

To determine your score, add all scores from the categories. Check your total score below to see if your health and your life are at risk. You may be referred to the risk-reducing nutrition plan, page 186, or the risk-reducing exercise plan, page 226.

0 to 8	**Low Risk**—Your risk of colon cancer is low because you are eating right and getting plenty of exercise. Keep eating a healthy diet, and your risk should remain low.
9 to 16	**Moderate Risk**—You have a moderate risk of developing colon cancer. You can improve your odds by exercising and following the risk-reducing nutrition plan.
17 to 24	**High Risk**—Your risk of colon cancer is high. You need to improve your diet by eating more complex carbohydrates and less fat—both saturated and unsaturated. Follow the risk-reducing nutrition plan, and make exercise a part of your daily life.
25+	**Very High Risk**—Your risk of colon cancer is very high. You can considerably lower your risk by following the risk-reducing nutrition plan and the risk-reducing exercise plan.

TAKE THIS TEST TO MEASURE YOUR
LUNG-CANCER RISK

This test measures your risk of developing lung cancer. Circle the score for each characteristic that applies to you. Total the score, then check your risk category on the opposite page.

Family History

Choose any that apply.
+5   Parent or close relative with lung cancer
+8   Parent or close relative with lung cancer, and you smoke cigarettes occasionally
+20   Parent or close relative with lung cancer, and you smoke cigarettes regularly

Smoking

Choose any that apply.

+8 You are a smoker (or you quit within the last 2 years), and you began smoking in your teens

+12 You are a smoker (or you quit within the last 2 years), and you have smoked for 20 years or more

+1 Smoke less than 1 pack of cigarettes a day

+3 Smoke about 1 pack of cigarettes a day

+4 Smoke about 1-1/2 packs of cigarettes a day

+5 Smoke 2 or more packs of cigarettes a day

+2 Smoke and inhale deeply

+1 Smoke marijuana once or twice a week

+2 Smoke marijuana almost every day

Environment

Choose any that apply.

+1 Live *or* work in a heavily air-polluted area

+2 Live *and* work in a heavily air-polluted area

+3 Live *or* work in a heavily air-polluted area *and* smoke cigarettes

+4 Live *and* work in a heavily air-polluted area *and* smoke cigarettes

+1 Live *or* work with smokers

+2 Live *and* work with smokers

+4 Exposed to asbestos in home or workplace

INTERPRETING YOUR SCORE

To determine your score, add all scores from the categories. Check your total score below to see if your health and your life are at risk.

0 to 8 **Low Risk**—Your risk of lung cancer is low.

9 to 12 **Moderate Risk**—You have a moderate risk of lung cancer. You can't change your heredity, but you can stop smoking.

13 to 20 **High Risk**—Your risk of lung cancer is high. Stop smoking now, avoid smoky places and you'll help lower your risk considerably.

21+ **Very High Risk**—Your risk of lung cancer is very high. Stop smoking now, avoid air-polluted or smoke-polluted places and you'll help lower your risk considerably.

TAKE THIS TEST TO MEASURE YOUR
PROSTATE-CANCER RISK

This test measures your risk of developing prostate cancer. Circle the score for each characteristic that applies to you. Total the score, then check your risk category on the opposite page.

Family History

Choose any that apply.

+2   Your father, uncle or brother had prostate cancer
+3   More than one close relative had prostate cancer
+1   You are black
−2   You are oriental

Diet

Choose any that apply.

+3   You eat whole-milk dairy products, such as cheese, butter, cream cheese and whole milk, every day or almost every day
+2   You eat fried or butter-sauce foods several times a week
+2   You eat pastries, ice cream or rich desserts at least several times a week
+2   You eat fatty meats, such as steak, hamburger, roast beef, sausage or cold cuts, almost every day
+2   You eat lots of butter, margarine or fried foods almost every day
+2   You eat high-fat, empty-calorie foods, such as chips, dips or French fries, several times a week

Personal

Choose any that apply.

+5   You took, or are taking, testosterone or androgen medications
+2   You are overweight by 20%
+3   You are overweight by more than 25%

INTERPRETING YOUR SCORE

To determine your score, add all scores from the categories. Check your total score below to see if your health and your life are at risk. You may be referred to the risk-reducing nutrition plan, page 186, or the permanent weight-loss program, page 204.

0 to 8	**Low Risk**—Your risk of prostate cancer is low, but don't overlook having an annual examination of the prostate gland if you are 40 or older.
9 to 15	**Moderate Risk**—Your risk of prostate cancer is moderate. Have an annual examination of the prostate gland if you are 40 or older.
16 to 22	**High Risk**—You are at high risk of developing prostate cancer. Have an examination of your prostate twice a year. Losing weight by following the permanent weight-loss diet will help lower your risk.
23 +	**Very High Risk**—You are at very high risk of developing prostate cancer. Have yearly or more-frequent prostate examinations. Lose weight with the permanent weight-loss diet, and follow the risk-reducing nutrition plan to help lower your risk.

*TAKE THIS TEST TO MEASURE YOUR
CERVICAL-CANCER RISK*

This test measures your risk of developing cervical cancer. Circle the score for each characteristic that applies to you. Total the score, then check your risk category on page 78.

Family History

Choose one.

   0   No history of cervical cancer in family

+1   Your mother, aunt, grandmother or sister had cervical cancer

Personal

Choose any that apply.

+ 3   You became sexually active before age 17
+ 1   You have had 2 sexual partners
+ 2   You have had 5 sexual partners
+ 3   You have had 6 to 10 sexual partners
+ 4   You have had more than 10 sexual partners
+ 3   You have had 2 or fewer sexual partners, but one of them has or had many sexual partners
+ 5   You have active or symptomless genital herpes
+ 3   You have, or had, genital warts or other viral infections
+ 5   You have had an abnormal Pap test
+ 1   You live or work with heavy smokers
+ 1   You took birth-control pills while you had persistent cervical dysplasia

Diet

Choose one.

0   You drink citrus juice or eat citrus fruit or other high-vitamin-C food every day.

+ 2   You do not drink citrus juice or eat citrus fruit or other high vitamin-C food every day

---

INTERPRETING YOUR SCORE

To determine your score, add all scores from the categories. Check your total score below to see if your health and your life are at risk.

0 to 8   **Low Risk**—Your risk of cervical cancer is low, but it's a good idea to have regular Pap tests.

9 to 12   **Moderate Risk**—You have a moderate risk of developing cervical cancer. Have regular Pap tests.

13 to 15   **High Risk**—Your risk of cervical cancer is high. See your gynecologist at least every 6 months for a Pap test.

16+   **Very High Risk**—Your risk of cervical cancer is very high. See your gynecologist every 6 months for a Pap test.

TAKE THIS TEST TO MEASURE YOUR
UTERINE-CANCER RISK

This test measures your risk of developing uterine (endometrial) cancer. Circle the score for each characteristic that applies to you. Total the score, then check your risk category on page 80.

Family History

Choose one.

   0   No family history of uterine cancer
+2   Your mother, aunt or sister had uterine cancer
+3   More than one close relative had uterine cancer

Personal

Choose any that apply.

+4   You took, or have been taking, estrogen replacement therapy for less than 5 years
+6   You took, or have been taking, estrogen replacement therapy for more than 5 years
−2   Your took, or have been taking, estrogen replacement *and* progestin
+2   You took the high-estrogen birth-control pill Oracen
−3   You took birth-control pills (other than Oracen) for 5 years or less
−4   You took birth-control pills (other than Oracen) for 5 to 10 years or longer
+3   You are overweight by 20%
+4   You are overweight by 30% or more
+1   You are diabetic
+1   You have high blood pressure
+1   You have or had uterine polyps
+3   You have never given birth
−2   You have had five or more children
+3   Your menopause began at age 50 or later
+2   You have had abnormal uterine bleeding
+1   You had Stein-Leventhal syndrome
+1   You had, or have, breast or ovarian cancer

INTERPRETING YOUR SCORE

To determine your score, add all scores from the categories. Check your total score below to see if your health and your life are at risk.

0 to 8   **Low Risk**—Your risk of uterine cancer is low, but don't overlook a yearly pelvic examination.

9 to 18   **Moderate Risk**—You have a moderate risk of uterine cancer; be sure to have a yearly pelvic examination.

19 to 25 **High Risk**—Your risk of uterine cancer is high. Consult your gynecologist about recommended diagnostic procedures and frequency of exams. Losing weight will help lower your risk.

26+   **Very High Risk**—Your risk of uterine cancer is very high. Consult your gynecologist about recommended diagnostic procedures and frequency of exams. Losing weight will help lower your risk.

TAKE THIS TEST TO MEASURE YOUR OVARIAN-CANCER RISK

This test measures your risk of developing ovarian cancer. Circle the score for each characteristic that applies to you. Total the score, then check your risk category on the opposite page.

Family History

Choose any that apply.
   +2   Your mother, aunt or sister had ovarian cancer
   +5   Two close relatives had ovarian cancer
   +8   More than two close relatives had ovarian cancer

Diet

Choose any that apply.
   +1   You eat fewer than 3 servings of fruit or vegetables a day
   +1   You do not eat an orange or deep-green fruit or vegetable every day

+1 You eat red meat more than you eat fish or poultry
+2 You eat animal fats, such as butter and lard, as opposed to vegetable fats, such as margarine or cooking oil

Personal

Choose any that apply.

+3 You use talcum powder on your genitals, diaphragm, sanitary pads or underwear
−2 You took birth-control pills for up to 5 years
−3 You took birth-control pills for more than 5 years
+1 You took, or are taking, estrogen-replacement therapy
+2 You have never given birth
−2 You had your first pregnancy before age 22
−2 You gave birth to more than five children

INTERPRETING YOUR SCORE

To determine your score, add all scores from the categories. Check your total score below to see if your health and your life are at risk. You may be referred to the risk-reducing nutrition plan, page 186.

0 to 8 **Low Risk**—Your risk of ovarian cancer is low, but a yearly gynecological exam is recommended.

9 to 12 **Moderate Risk**—Your risk of ovarian cancer is moderate, but a yearly gynecological exam is recommended.

13 to 15 **High Risk**—You have a high risk of ovarian cancer. Report any unusual gastrointestinal symptoms, such as continual gassiness, abdominal pressure, fullness, heartburn or belching, to your gynecologist immediately. You can help reduce your risk by following the risk-reducing nutrition plan.

16+ **Very High Risk**—You have a very high risk of getting ovarian cancer. Report any unusual gastrointestinal symptoms, such as continual gassiness, abdominal pressure, fullness, heartburn or belching, to your gynecologist immediately. You can help reduce your risk by following the risk-reducing nutrition plan.

TAKE THIS TEST TO MEASURE YOUR
SKIN-CANCER AND MELANOMA RISK

This test measures your risk of developing skin cancer (basal-cell and squamous-cell) and malignant melanoma. Circle the score for each characteristic that applies to you. Total the score, then check your risk on opposite page.

Family History

Choose any that apply.

+8   Parent or close relative with malignant melanoma
+10 Parent or close relative with melanoma, and you have a pigmented mole

Personal

Choose any that apply.

+4   Always burn easily and severely, tan little or not at all, and peel when burned
+3   Usually burn easily and severely, tan lightly but often peel
+2   Burn moderately and tan moderately
+1   Burn minimally, tan easily and more darkly with each exposure
−2   Burn rarely; tan easily and deeply
−3   Never burn; tan deeply
+2   Unexposed skin is white
−1   Unexposed skin is light brown
−3   Unexposed skin is black
+3   Have light complexion with blue or light-colored eyes
+2   Have a light complexion with brown or dark eyes
+2   Have light complexion, dark hair and freckles
+3   Have a light complexion, blond or red hair and freckles
+3   Have a mole larger than a dime
+3   Have an obvious mole that was present at birth
+10 Have a mole with very dark or irregular borders or pigment patterns

Sun Exposure

Choose any that apply.

+3   Live in low-latitude or high-altitude area
+2   Try to achieve a tan every summer or vacation

+1   Work or spend considerable time outdoors
+3   Vacation in strong sunlight, such as in the tropics, desert or mountains, and get regular sun exposure at home
+6   Vacation in strong sunlight, such as in the tropics, desert or mountains, but otherwise do not get much regular sun exposure at home
+3   Exposed to strong sun on the weekends but not during the week
+6   Experienced one severe, blistering sunburn as a child
+10 Experienced more than one blistering sunburn as a child
+3   Experienced severe sunburns as an adult
−5   Always apply sunscreen (SPF 15) before spending time in the sun

---

INTERPRETING YOUR SCORE

To determine your score, add all scores from the categories. Check your total score below to see if your health and your life are at risk.

0 to 10   **Low Risk**—Your risk of skin cancer and melanoma is low because you tan readily and easily and are not overly exposed to the sun.

11 to 20 **Moderate Risk**—You have a moderate risk of developing skin cancer or melanoma because you are exposed infrequently to strong sunlight and may get a sunburn. Moderate your sun exposure, avoid the hottest times of the day and use sunscreen before you begin to burn.

21 to 30 **High Risk**—You have a high risk of developing skin cancer because you have sun-sensitive skin and are over-exposed to the sun. Use a powerful sunscreen (SPF 15), and wear a hat when you are in the sun. Avoid being in the sun during the hottest times of the day. Report any changes in your skin or moles to your doctor immediately.

31+   **Very High Risk**—You have a very high risk of developing skin cancer or melanoma because you have sun-sensitive skin and are overexposed to damaging sunlight. Limit your time in strong sunlight, use a powerful sunscreen (SPF 15) and wear a hat when outdoors in the sun. Report any changes in your skin or moles to your doctor immediately.

TAKE THIS TEST TO MEASURE YOUR GASTROINTESTINAL-CANCER RISK

This test measures your risk of developing gastrointestinal-tract (GI) cancer. Circle the score for each characteristic that applies to you. Total the score, then check your risk category on the opposite page.

Family History

Choose any that apply.

+ 8   One or more relatives with cancer of the stomach or esophagus, and you smoke and drink

+ 3   One or more close relative with pancreatic cancer, and you drink more than 2 cups of coffee a day

Diet

Choose any that apply.

+ 3   Eat large quantities of pickled foods more than 3 times a week

+ 1   Eat processed meats containing nitrate or nitrite, such as bacon, sausage, cold cuts and hot dogs, once a week

+ 3   Eat processed meats containing nitrate or nitrite, such as bacon, sausage, cold cuts and hot dogs, 2 or 3 times a week

+ 4   Eat processed meats containing nitrate or nitrite, such as bacon, sausage, cold cuts and hot dogs, almost every day

+ 1   Eat smoked or barbecued food once a week

+ 2   Eat smoked or barbecued food several times a week

+ 4   Eat smoked or barbecued food almost every day

+ 2   Eat whole-milk dairy products, such as cheese, butter, cream cheese, ice cream or whole milk, every day

+ 2   Eat fried or butter-sauce foods several times a week

+ 3   Eat generous portions of margarine or salad dressings every day

+ 2   Eat pastries or rich desserts several times a week

+ 4   Eat meat every day

− 3   Eat at least 3 servings of fruits and vegetables every day

Smoking and Chemicals

Choose any that apply.

+ 4   Smoke 1 or more packs of cigarettes a day

+ 8   Smoke 1 or more packs of cigarettes a day and drink more than two 5-ounce glasses of wine or 12-ounce glasses of beer or 3 ounces of hard liquor a day

+6   Smoke 1 or more packs of cigarettes a day and work with dangerous chemicals, such as pesticides

+2   You have been exposed to industrial chemicals, such as beta-naphthalene, benzidine or urea

Personal

Choose any that apply.

+2   You are black

+2   You are male

INTERPRETING YOUR SCORE

To determine your score, add all scores from the categories. Check your total score below to see if your health and your life are at risk. You may be referred to the risk-reducing nutrition plan, page 186.

0 to 10   **Low Risk**—Your risk of pancreatic, stomach or esophagal cancer is low. Keep up the good dietary and smoking habits, and your risk should remain negligible.

11 to 19   **Moderate Risk**—You have a moderate risk of developing cancer of the stomach, pancreas or esophagus. Eat a low-fat, low-protein diet, stop smoking and reduce your alcohol consumption to help decrease your risks.

20 to 30   **High Risk**—Your risk of developing stomach, pancreas or esophagal cancer is high. Take steps *now* to help reduce the fat and protein in your diet. Stop smoking, and cut down on alcohol.

31+   **Very High Risk**—Your risk of developing stomach, pancreas or esophagal cancer is very high. Begin the risk-reducing nutrition plan, stop smoking and drink moderately, and you'll help lower your risk considerably.

The Major Risk Factors of Cancer

Cancer is a real threat for nearly every North American. Though heart disease is the greater killer, the possibility of being stricken with cancer is real for many people. Each year, approximately 850,000 new cases of life-threatening cancers are diagnosed in the United States; 440,000 die from cancer. Lung cancer is the leading culprit, with 145,000 new cases and 125,000 deaths each year. Close behind, and becoming more frequent every year, is colon cancer, which strikes 140,000 people each year and causes 60,000 deaths. Breast cancer strikes 120,000 people (mostly women), causing 39,000 deaths; prostate cancer accounts for 86,000 cases with 25,000 deaths each year. Many of these cancers are rising steadily in frequency among the American people. See illustration on opposite page.

Why this rise in cancers? The answer lies not in chemical pollutants, food additives or nuclear contaminants, where much of our concern is focused, but in our lifestyle. Researchers believe that as much as 75% of all cancers are the result of improper diet, tobacco use and heavy alcohol consumption. Cigarette smoking causes more than 75% of all cases of lung cancer—83% of those in men and 45% of those in women. The lung-cancer rate among women is rising because of increased smoking among women. A high-fat, low-fiber diet is a major cause of breast cancer and colon cancer. Heavy alcohol consumption, together with cigarette smoking, plays a major role in gastrointestinal cancer and cancers of the esophagus and the pancreas. Overexposure to the sun, through sunbathing or working unprotected outdoors, causes most of the malignant melanomas, another steadily increasing cancer.

Who you are—male, female, black, white—and where you live—East, West, North, South—is no bar to cancer. You aren't safe from your own bad habits!

WHAT CAUSES CANCER?

Scientists' understanding of what causes cancer has increased because of decades of painstaking research. Cancer is not really a single disease with a single cause; different forms of cancer are caused by many different stimuli.

All cancers begin on a molecular level within the cells. Every cell in your body contains smaller structures that carry out the cell's functions. If a cell receives cancer-promoting stimulus from a virus, radiation, hormone imbalance, a noxious element (such as in tobacco smoke or the aflatoxin in moldy peanuts) or any of a multitude of other suspected carcinogenic agents, the affected cell begins to grow abnormally. Many researchers believe all of us at some time have changes in our cells that make them potentially cancerous. However, the immune system's normal mechanisms almost always react immediately to wipe out these precancerous cells.

There are 46 chromosomes in the nucleus of every cell; these carry the genetic

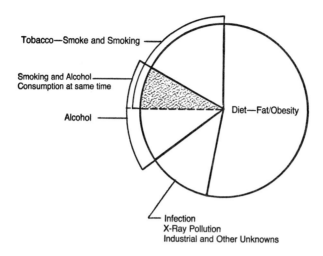

Causes of cancer in the United States. Based on data from the National Center for Health Statistics.

material that serves as the body's blueprint. Chromosomes are composed of sub-groups of molecules called *genes,* which contain the instructions on how a cell should grow. There are an estimated 200 or more genes on each of these 46 chromosomes. It is in the genes where cancer begins; it starts as a mutation or change in the genes' molecules. The nucleic acids—DNA—that are the genes' building blocks may become damaged or rearranged (mutated) so that as the cells multiply and grow, they do so along malignant pathways.

The real danger of cancer may begin when your anti-cancer mechanism is neutral-ized or rendered impotent by one of many mechanisms, and precancerous cells are not routinely wiped out. This may happen when there is not enough fiber in your diet, leaving cancer-promoting elements in the intestine to proceed unhindered. Or your immune system may become weakened by a poor diet or by an overwhelming bombardment of infectious viral, bacterial or other agents and become unable to maintain its cancer-preventive action.

These explanations of present cancer theories are overly simplified. The checks and balances within your body are extremely complex, and medical researchers are still a long way from understanding all the complexities.

Though our knowledge of cancer's exact biological mechanisms remains in-complete, you can take advantage of current knowledge to reduce your risk of malignancy. Take the various cancer risk-factor tests at the beginning of this section to measure your susceptibility to cancer, then read on to discover what you can do to lower your risks.

Most of the cancer risk factors I discuss are choices you make for yourself, so it seems imperative that if you find yourself at high risk, you need to change your ways. This probably means changing your diet, stopping smoking and getting more exercise. Certain foods can help *protect* you from cancer. You can take positive measures to help lower your risk of cancer by following the risk-reducing nutrition plan, page 186, and the risk-reducing exercise plan, page 226. You don't have to be one of the grim statistics if you change your ways.

THE FAT RISK FACTOR

It has been well-documented that populations consuming a high proportion of their diet as fat have a much higher occurrence of cancer than population groups that eat much less fat. The "epidemic" of cancers seems to show up in populations where 40% or more of the calories in the diet come from fat.

Our diet typically contains 40% fat. The fat comes from butter, margarine, cooking oil, hamburger, steak, chicken skin, chocolate cake, whole milk and many other foods. Although it is a nutritious source of protein, calcium and vitamins, a glass of whole milk, which is only 3-1/2% fat by volume, contains 45% of its calories in that fat. Skim milk offers the same nutrition but *without* the fat.

Fat molecules are rich in single-oxygen molecules and free radicals (charged particles), both of which are chemically very active. Many researchers believe oxidized fats (fats that have undergone chemical reactions) are carcinogenic (cancer-producing) agents. Under normal circumstances, these reactive molecules are neutralized by your body's natural biochemical reactions. If viruses, X-rays or other carcinogenic chemicals invade the cells, chemical changes may get out of control, damaging your cell's DNA so cells take a pathway toward malignant growth.

Cancer of the colon, which follows cancers of the lung in number of reported cases a year, is rapidly increasing in incidence. As our population ages, our poor lifestyle and improper eating habits have time to catch up, making themselves known by the increased national rate of colon cancer. This type of cancer is linked to the amount of fat in the diet. The fat can be any kind—saturated or unsaturated, animal or vegetable. While it is not thoroughly established how dietary fat causes cancer, researchers theorize excess fat in the intestinal tract negates the natural anti-cancer mechanism.

If you eat a diet high in fat, your liver will produce more of a particular fat called *sterol*. Sterol enters the small intestine with bile from the liver and induces an increase in the production of bile acids. An increase in bile acids results in an increase in the bowel bacteria that metabolize the bile into cancer-promoting bile salts. A diet high in fat and low in fiber allows for an increase in the concentration of the bile acid and carcinogens in the colon.

Cancer of the colon is virtually unknown in primitive cultures, where diets are low in fat and high in fiber. Rice, vegetables and grains are eaten whole and unprocessed in many African populations, and these people have almost no incidence of colon cancer. The fiber in these foods is not digested by intestinal enzymes; it binds water in the intestinal tract, increasing stool bulk and volume. At the same time, fiber dilutes potential carcinogens. Any carcinogens present pass through the colon more quickly (this type of diet encourages frequent bowel movements) and will not linger in contact with the colon wall.

Colon carcinoma occurs with high frequency where beef is the source of fat. This is seen in data gathered from around the world. Populations that eat the highest amount of beef per capita—New Zealand, Argentina, Uruguay and the United States—have significantly higher rates of colon cancer than countries where beef consumption is low. The highest rate of this disease occurs in New Zealand, where people eat more beef than anywhere else in the world.

According to the National Research Council, vegetarian Adventists, who eat 25% less fat and 50% more fiber than the average American, have a very low incidence of colon carcinoma. Those who do not adhere strictly to their dietary customs have an increased rate of colon cancer in proportion to the amount of beef they eat. Mormons, who eat a lot of beef but who don't smoke or drink, have an incidence midway between Adventists and the general population. This suggests smoking and alcohol have an additive effect in inducing cancer in the presence of a high-fat diet.

Colon cancer is not the only type of cancer induced by a high-fat diet. Breast cancer and uterine cancer also have an association with a fatty diet. Cancer researchers suspect obesity is a risk factor for endometrial cancer and breast cancer in post-menopausal women.

The rate of breast cancer in Japanese women, who consume a diet characteristically low in fat, is 1/6 that of women in the United States. But second-generation Japanese women living in Hawaii have a breast-cancer rate equal to the overall American population, suggesting diet and living habits, not an inherent genetic protection, account for the low cancer rate in Japan.

In the United States, vegetarian women have a much lower breast-cancer rate. The mortality rate from breast cancer in the United States is 6 times higher than Asian and African populations. As with colon cancer, the highest correlation among all variables in the populations studied was total dietary fat.

The presence of extra amounts of dietary fat causes the liver to convert naturally occurring androgens (male hormones) in a woman's body into estrogen. This excess estrogen leads to greater estrogen stimulation of the breast and uterus. The more prolonged the stimulus, the greater the chances of cancer.

Prostate cancer is a risk for men who eat a high-fat diet. The increased estrogen in their systems, which results from excess dietary fat, results in increased androgen receptors in the prostate. The increased stimulation of the prostate by androgens can promote cancer. An unfortunate result of a high-fat diet is that the increased estrogen-to-androgen ratio reduces a man's sexual potency.

ARE YOUR EMOTIONS A RISK FACTOR?

Research involving how emotions and stress affect the incidence of cancer is a growing new field. Some people may have cancer-prone personalities. A recent report from epidemiologists at the California Department of Health Services in Berkeley reveals emotions may play an important role in development of cancer. They followed nearly 7,000 people for 17 years to see who would develop cancer. The results showed women who felt socially isolated and had few social contacts had a 500% greater risk of dying from breast and lymph cancer than women who had many social contacts and did not feel isolated. Women who had few social contacts, but who did not report feeling isolated, had 500% greater rate of developing lung cancer.

How feelings and life situations affect cancer remains to be seen. Hormones from stress and other emotions may repeatedly challenge the body's immune system, eventually allowing a precancerous cell to escape and begin a malignant growth.

YOUR NEED TO EXERCISE

Research by Dr. David Garabrant at the University of Southern California shows that sedentary men are 60% more likely to get colon cancer than men whose jobs require physical activity. This is probably because exercise helps fight constipation, shortening the time potential cancer-causing agents spend in the bowel.

The 10-year-long study of 17,000 Harvard alumni men directed by Dr. Ralph Paffenberger at the Stanford University Medical Center revealed some surprising results. The men who were most physically active, especially those who participated in vigorous activities, had a lower death rate from cancer, as well as from heart disease and all other causes.

CAN FOOD ADDITIVES CAUSE CANCER?

If you read labels on packaged or prepared food, you may be struck by the extensive list of chemicals among the ingredients. Most of these compounds are harmless and are actually the biochemical names for natural food substances. But certain compounds are implicated in causing cancer, and you should avoid them. Read labels!

Preservatives are added to a food to keep it from spoiling. Oils, cereals and flour-based products frequently have BHT and BHA added to them. These compounds pose no danger and may actually be protective against cancer because they prevent the oxidation of fats into cancer-causing agents.

Be cautious about food containing nitrate or nitrite compounds. These preservatives are added to meat products, such as ham, bacon and luncheon meat, to maintain the red color and to prevent the growth of the botulism bacteria. Botulism bacteria gives off a tasteless, highly toxic poison that causes food poisoning and frequently death. Scientists believe the risk of cancer is preferable to the risk of food poisoning, so the FDA has not banned these compounds. However, it lowered the allowable quantity of the compounds to safer levels. The food industry has almost eliminated the use of nitrate, which is a more serious health threat than nitrite. Nitrate and nitrite compounds can change into carcinogenic compounds in your digestive system. It may seem like a trade-off whether to allow these compounds in foods at all.

Inside the stomach, nitrates and nitrites combine with the breakdown products of protein to form nitrosamines. Nitrosamine compounds have a strong carcinogenic potential. If you eat foods with these chemicals, it's wise to read labels closely. Choose brands that also list ascorbic acid (vitamin C) as an ingredient—ascorbic acid is an anti-oxidant and prevents formation of nitrosamines.

Other chemicals are frequently used in food preparation. Cyclamate, saccharin and aspartame are chemicals that taste sweet but have no calories because they can't be digested. Cyclamate and saccharin were once widely used as artificial sweeteners, but the FDA banned cyclamate when it came under suspicion in causing certain kinds of cancer, particularly bladder cancer. Because of public demand, saccharin is still used, but it also is a cancer-causing suspect. In large doses, it causes cancer in laboratory rats.

The newest artificial sweetener is aspartame, sold under the brand names Nutra-sweet and Equal. It has been touted as a safe additive because it is made from natural ingredients. It remains to be seen if this sweetener will follow the same course as other artificial sweeteners. Some researchers believe aspartame may stimulate the carbohydrate-craving mechanism in the brain, increasing your craving for sweets. This may offset any weight-loss effort you may be attempting.

The real problem with artificial sweeteners is not that they are strong carcinogens themselves, but that they are cancer "promoters." A promoter is a chemical substance that does not cause cancer but promotes and speeds the growth of cancer cells already present. In effect, a promoter acts together with other carcinogens to make them much more insidious!

Unassailable evidence of the danger of artificial sweeteners has not yet been demonstrated, but why take the risk? Artificial sweeteners are not a necessary food item, so it may be wise to avoid them. An occasional diet soft drink won't do much harm, but daily use of artificial sweeteners in coffee, tea or diet soft drinks may expose you to a harmful amount of these additives.

Some researchers have expressed concern over smoked and barbecued foods. The

91

incidence of stomach cancer has steadily decreased in the United States, but it is alarmingly high in Iceland. Studies suggest their diet, which consists of large quantities of smoked fish and other smoked foods, is a causative factor because the smoking process produces polycyclic aromatic hydrocarbons in the food. Hydrocarbons are known to cause cancer. Charcoal-grilling and barbecuing meats may also produce hydrocarbons because as the fat drips from the meat onto the hot coals it smokes, coating the outside of the meat with hydrocarbons.

The incidence of stomach cancer has been decreasing, so researchers have paid less attention to smoking and charcoal-grilling as possible causes of cancer. But if these methods of food preparation are risky, the quantity of the foods and the frequency with which you eat them is a major consideration. I would not suggest you eliminate all smoked or barbecued foods if you enjoy them, but it might be best to limit your consumption to only once a week so exposure to hydrocarbons is not great.

IS COFFEE A HAZARD?

Two separate research studies, one from Harvard University and one from Johns Hopkins University, report an apparent association between high coffee consumption and pancreatic cancer. It didn't seem to make any difference whether the coffee was caffeinated or decaffeinated—the same association was statistically present. Though more research needs to be done to reach a final conclusion, these studies cannot be ignored.

If your family has a history of pancreatic cancer, you may be susceptible to the disease, so limit your coffee consumption. The frequency and quantity of coffee you drink are key risk factors of this cancer. You don't need to give up drinking coffee entirely, but limit your consumption to one or two cups a day.

Caffeinated coffee has also been implicated as a factor in development of pain in the breasts. Caffeine and related theobromine compounds from coffee, tea, cola and chocolate can cause a fibrocystic condition of the breast. This is a benign condition, but women who have this problem may have an increased incidence of breast cancer when compared with women who do not have fibrocystic disease. If you have a fibrocystic condition, it may be wise to reduce your caffeine consumption.

THE SMOKING RISK FACTOR

The role cigarette smoking plays in lung cancer is notorious—smoking accounts for 75% of all lung cancer, the cancer of greatest frequency in this country. After you have smoked 7,000 to 10,000 cigarettes a year for several years (a pack a day), the cells lining the bronchial walls become damaged and allow precancerous cells to begin their malignant growth.

In a healthy person, the body's immune system constantly defends the body against such cells. In smokers, the activity of these "natural killer cells" diminishes. Genetic factors may be at work so that on the average, a smoker is *10 times* more likely to get lung cancer than a non-smoker. The child of a person who smoked and suffered from lung cancer is *15 to 25 times* more likely to get lung cancer if he smokes than if he does not smoke.

According to the National Centers for Disease Control, lung cancer has become a leading killer among women. Its incidence has even surpassed breast cancer in several places. This is because women and teenage girls smoke now more than ever before, and smoking puts their lungs and hearts at risk.

The damage caused by cigarette smoking doesn't stop with lung cancer. Smoking is associated with cancers of the esophagus, stomach and pancreas. If smoking is combined with regular, heavy consumption of alcohol, there is a combined effect on the upper gastrointestinal tract, which dramatically increases the likelihood of esophagal and pancreatic cancer. A recent study showed women who do not smoke, but who live with smokers, are at greater risk of cervical and breast cancer, though the reason for this is unclear.

If you currently smoke, drink alcohol in excess and eat a high-fat, low-fiber diet, you are at highest risk of developing several different types of cancer. You can change your lifestyle to help you lower risks.

ARE HORMONES A RISK FACTOR?

During the '50s and '60s, and even into the early '70s, the estrogenlike hormone DES (diethystilbestrol) was given to pregnant women to prevent miscarriage. This seemingly harmless compound has caused many tragedies—many girls born to DES mothers developed a rare form of vaginal cancer in their teens or 20s. If you know your mother took DES while she was pregnant with you, you should be under close observation by your doctor. He will be able to identify early signs of cancer before it becomes life-threatening.

A recent report of research done at Dartmouth College, which followed more than 6,000 women who took DES during pregnancy, showed those women were at increased risk of breast cancer; they had a 41% higher risk of breast cancer when compared to women who had not taken DES. The effect of the DES takes almost 20 years to manifest itself.

Not long ago, DES was fed to cattle to help them gain weight. Although the amount you would receive from eating meat of DES-fed animals is extremely low and not likely to cause disease, it is no longer legal to feed DES to livestock because the compound has been demonstrated to be a carcinogenic agent.

After more than 20 years of concern regarding the safety of birth-control pills, which contain estrogen and progesterone, it now appears fear of the pill causing cancer was unwarranted. Statistics actually suggest a *decrease* in the incidence of uterine and ovarian cancer among pill users and former pill users. Pill users have the same incidence of breast cancer as non-users. Although the pill does not cause cancer, it can cause serious vascular and metabolic complications, especially in women who smoke.

Women frequently take estrogen when they begin to experience the symptoms of menopause. The hormone is used to replace the naturally falling estrogen levels in their bodies. Estrogen replacement reduces many unpleasant effects of menopause, such as hot flashes and vaginal dryness. Some medical researchers believe it also helps protect the bones from losing calcium, thus preventing osteoporosis.

Continued long-term use of estrogen replacement in post-menopausal women increases the risk of developing cancer in the lining of the uterine wall (endometrium). While the incidence of this disease is less than it was believed to be 10 years ago, a measurable risk does exist. Estrogen-replacement therapy also causes an increased risk of heart disease and stroke.

Many gynecologists today prescribe a regimen that combines estrogen and progesterone, in hopes of gaining the same protection as that provided by the combination of these hormones in birth-control pills. This combination provides protection from endometrial cancer, but its effects on heart disease and stroke are unknown. Whether the benefits of estrogen-replacement therapy outweigh the risks is an individual matter that should be decided between a woman and her gynecologist.

YOUR RISK OF BREAST CANCER

The incidence of breast cancer in American women has increased steadily in the last 40 years. Today, 9% of all American women will develop the disease. A high-fat diet may be the primary cause of breast cancer, but a woman's reproductive history also plays a part.

The lowest incidence of breast cancer occurs in women who gave birth before age 20. The highest rate occurs among women who never bore a child. Those who have their first child after 35 have a rate similar to that of childless women. Women who breast-fed their babies have the same rate of breast cancer as women who did not.

There seems to be a genetic susceptibility toward breast cancer; a mother or sister with breast cancer is your *most serious* risk factor of developing the disease. Lifestyle similarities—especially the same high-fat diet—may be the cause of this family history rather than an actual genetic cause. But for whatever reason, the family link is significant.

The use of X-ray exams (mammograms) to detect breast cancer was once considered to pose a small risk of developing the disease because overexposure to X-rays can cause cancer. But the amount of radiation used in mammography has been sharply reduced—from 8 rads to 1 rad or less, and the risk is now considered to be minimal. Mammography is highly effective in diagnosing breast cancer, even before a lump can be felt, so *all* women at high risk should have regular mammograms.

The American Cancer Society recommends the following guidelines. In addition to regular monthly self-examinations, a woman should:

- Have a baseline mammogram between ages 35 and 40.
- Have a mammogram once every 1 or 2 years between ages 40 and 45.
- Have a yearly mammogram after age 50.
- Consult her physician about need for more-frequent mammograms if she has a family history of breast cancer.

IS THE HERPES VIRUS RELATED TO CANCER?

The herpes virus may be one cause of cervical cancer. The frequency of herpes infection has been explosive during the past 10 years, while the frequency of cervical cancer has declined over the past 20 years, but the virus is still suspect.

Herpes simplex I, the common cold-sore virus, and herpes zoster, the virus of shingles, do not appear to be cancer causing. People who have cancer develop shingles easily, but that's because their immune systems are already weakened.

The herpes viruses of the sexual organs, herpes simplex II and occasionally herpes simplex I (transmitted from non-sexual areas to the genitals) are suspect as cancer-producing agents. This viral infection is transmitted from person to person by lesions that are moist and secrete fluids. The virus is not contagious when lesions have dried up or are not present. Treatment for herpes is available, but no cure or vaccine has been developed.

If you have herpes, the risk of cervical cancer is very low. If you suffer from herpes, it would be wise to have yearly Pap tests, which can detect cervical cancer before it spreads.

Cervical cancer is more common in women who have had several sexual partners or whose partner has had many different partners. Sexual intercourse beginning at age 16 or younger also increases the risk. These factors indicate some transmittable agent other than herpes virus may also be involved.

ULTRAVIOLET LIGHT AND THE RISK OF SKIN CANCER

Sunlight consists of ultraviolet (UV) and infrared waves. UV light is a powerful mutagen, causing mutations in your cell's genetic material. In fact, UV light is used in laboratory tests to cause mutation in bacteria and other microorganisms. Dark-pigmented or tanned skin helps slow damage from ultraviolet rays, but in unprotected skin, the genetic material within the skin cells absorbs ultraviolet light and may cause a mutation. If the cell's normal repair mechanisms fail to repair the mutation, the cell could go on to produce a cancer cell. Tanned or dark skin can withstand more sun than light skin, but dark skin *can* be damaged by overexposure to sunlight. Like light skin, dark or tanned skin can burn, but the burn may not be visible.

Infrared light, which is one of the rays of solar light, may also cause premalignant change in the epidermis. Sun lamps and tanning salons, which use various types of ultraviolet light, may produce cancer when used excessively.

People most susceptible to UV damage have a light complexion, light-colored eyes, blond or red hair and freckles; they burn easily and tan poorly. People with skin diseases, particularly pigmented diseases of the skin, and those whose skin is more lucent, are also at high risk of skin cancer. Anyone who freckles easily has an impaired mechanism for repairing damaged DNA in skin cells and is at highest risk. In any skin type, too much sun increases your risk of skin cancer and premature wrinkling of the skin.

Basal-cell, squamous-cell and malignant-melanoma cancers are induced primarily by overexposure to ultraviolet light. The amount of exposure has a cumulative effect—the more you're exposed, the greater your chances of developing skin cancer. Severe sunburns in young children are related to later development of skin cancer.

In the United States, the highest rate of skin cancer occurs in the Southwest where the low latitude or high altitude and love of the outdoors means people are exposed excessively to ultraviolet light.

The incidence of malignant melanoma, a deadly cancer that begins in the skin's pigment cells, has risen alarmingly in recent years. Researchers attribute this to our quests for a tan and to the growing number of people living in the Sunbelt area. Malignant melanoma most commonly strikes people who get intermittent exposure to strong sun, such as only on weekends or during yearly vacations.

Melanoma occurs more frequently in people who have pigmented moles. If you have a relative with melanoma, your chance of developing the cancer increases 8 times.

You can protect yourself from skin cancer. Don't be a sun-worshipper. A deep tan may be becoming, but it causes premature aging and drying of the skin and may lead to skin cancer. Protect yourself from the sun's harmful rays by wearing sunscreen containing PABA when you are outside in strong sun, especially if you are in a high-risk group.

Sunscreens are rated according to their ability to protect your skin from burning. The higher the rating number, the stronger the protection. If you're in a high-risk group, use SPF 15 sunscreen; reapply it frequently if you swim or perspire.

Avoid midday sun, and be aware that sand, water and snow reflect light, even on overcast days, increasing the strength of the sun. Ordinary window glass filters out UV light; it's best to use sunglasses made from safety glass rather than plastic or have glasses treated with an ultraviolet-filtering coating. Wearing a hat adds further protection.

RADIATION AND THE RISK OF CANCER

Radiation can cause cancer, but in our daily lives, few of us are exposed to enough radiation to cause worry. Radiation damages DNA in the genetic material in biological cells, much in the same way as UV light does, but radiation can penetrate deep into the body. Human cells can tolerate a small amount of radiation because part of a cell's normal function is to repair damage to DNA. When exposure goes above the safe threshold, the repair mechanisms can't keep up with the damage, and a malignancy can result. In Japanese who were exposed to radiation of the atomic bomb, there is a high incidence of malignancy of organs especially sensitive to radiation, such as blood-forming organs, bone marrow, thymus and thyroid.

Frequent exposure to diagnostic medical and X-ray procedures may exceed the safety threshold. Keep your doctor informed of any X-ray procedures you have had. The risk of any diagnostic X-rays required should be gauged by your physician against the importance of the information to be gained.

Newer forms of diagnostic examinations, such as ultrasound and MR (magnetic resonance), are now being used to provide information similar to X-rays, and they don't expose you to radiation. When possible, choose these forms of diagnosis rather than standard X-rays.

ENVIRONMENTAL POLLUTANTS AND THE RISK OF CANCER

The publicity given to environmental chemical pollutants, such as PCB, EDB and dioxin, has created an epidemic of fear among the public and has led people to assume that chemical pollutants are responsible for the majority of cancers. Evidence is to the contrary! Chemical pollutants *can* cause cancer, but according to the National Cancer Institute and the U.S. Public Health Service, it seems likely these chemicals are responsible for *only* 4 to 8% of *all* cancers. Nevertheless, this accounts for many thousands of deaths—unnecessary ones.

The evidence against chemicals in the environment and in our food indicts only 166 chemicals among the thousands commonly used in industry and the home. Of these, only 22 are proven carcinogenic, but another 94 are suspect. Asbestos is the worst chemical, according to a 1982 report from the National Toxicity Program; it has caused more cancer deaths than all other carcinogens combined.

Some chemical carcinogens are described on the following page. Chemicals that have been banned and removed from the market, such as TRIS (the fire-retardent once applied to children's clothing), are not included.

Within your own home and workplace, make every effort to avoid exposure to carcinogenic agents. Chemical industries in your region may be disposing of waste products, either in the air or in the water. Construction of new buildings may be

Chemical	Where Found	Who's at Risk
Arsenic	Used in pesticides, paints and wood preservatives. A byproduct of copper and lead smelting. Air, water and food contaminant.	Workers at smelting and pesticide plants. People living in vicinity of such plants.
Asbestos	Used in fireproofing and insulation products, wallboard, brake linings, caulking, roofing and flooring. Air pollutant; may be absorbed by the skin.	Mining, milling, manufacturing and construction workers. School children in deteriorating schools.
Benzene	Raw material in rubber, chemical and drug industries. Used in gasoline, adhesives, pesticides, inks and paint. Emissions from oil and coke refineries. Exposure by ingestion, skin absorption or inhalation.	Most of population is exposed to low levels. Highest exposure at gas stations, in urban areas and among workers at refineries.
EDB	Chemical in pesticides and leaded gasoline. Absorbed by the skin and inhalation.	Exposure in food and air for most of the population.
Formaldehyde	Gas often dissolved in water as formalin. Used in plastics, building materials, foam insulation, embalming fluid, soil fumigants, room deodorants and cosmetics. Exposure by inhalation and skin absorption.	Beauticians, morticians and pesticide workers, workers in manufacturing plants and people living nearby.
Hair Dye	The chemical 4-methoxy-m-phynelenediamine (4-MMPD) used in permanent hair dyes. Absorption by the skin.	Women and men who use or apply hair dye containing 4-MMPD.
Nickel	Used as a metal alloy in ship-building, aerospace and other heavy industry. Air and water pollutant.	Entire population exposed to low levels. Workers in industry and those living near manufacturing plants.
PCB	A banned chemical still persistent in the environment. Used in electrical industry and pesticides. Water, soil and air contaminant.	Entire population is exposed to low levels. Highest exposure comes from contaminated water and from living near incinerator sites.
Vinyl Chloride	Gaseous raw material used in plastics and floor tiles. Now banned from plastic food wrap and plastic beverage bottles.	Industrial workers. People who frequently used aerosol-propellant sprays.

distributing invisible asbestos into the air. Your constant vigilance of local newspapers and communication with the local Board of Health may give you clues to possible exposure. Be vigilant but not hysterical about your environment.

Some researchers have shown air inside a house can be more dangerous than the air outside, even in air-polluted areas. Fumes from household chemicals, paints, glues and cigarette smoke build up and are trapped by well-insulated structures. Formaldehye-containing chemicals and household items, such as air fresheners and pressed board, should be avoided. It's imperative to ventilate your house well when working with any chemical-based product. If anyone in your home smokes, air out the house regularly to get rid of noxious fumes.

Asbestos can be a risk at home, in the workplace or at school because it was frequently used to insulate heating and cooling ducts. Check to see if ducts are asbestos lined. Request to have asbestos removed at schools and your workplace. At home, have it removed by an experienced professional, especially if the asbestos is crumbling or deteriorating. Careless removal may leave behind many microscopic particles, making the situation worse than before.

Cigarette smoking compounds your risk of asbestos-related cancers. People who were exposed to asbestos, such as shipbuilders, who also smoke have a cancer risk 20 times higher than people who were exposed but never smoked. If you've been exposed to asbestos, there's little you can do about it—but you can stop smoking!

We frequently feel helpless to control chemical pollutants that threaten our health, but fortunately dangers are less alarming than we once believed. The biggest step you can take to lower your risk of environmentally caused cancer is to use a sunscreen if you are fair-complexioned, reduce your exposure to intense sunshine, use chemicals wisely, get plenty of fresh air and stop smoking!

8.

LOWER YOUR RISK OF CANCER

At some time, 25% of all North Americans will contract cancer! No one can guarantee who will and who will not get cancer because the disease often develops slowly over several decades before it manifests itself. But if you begin taking certain precautions *now,* you may considerably reduce your risk of cancer. Cancer experts believe between 65 and 90% of all cancer cases in this country need not occur—they result from lifestyle choices that are yours to make.

STOP SMOKING NOW!

Tobacco smoke is the *most serious* carcinogenic agent we are exposed to on a regular basis. Smoke from tobacco is a potent carcinogen that produces deadly cancers where there otherwise would not have been any disease. Thirty percent of all cancers probably come from tobacco use—280,000 cases a year that don't have to be! Twenty percent of all teenagers and 30% of all adults in this country smoke, and they expose non-smoking people to the noxious fumes.

If you smoke, stop now! It's difficult, but with the proper help you can do it. If you can't stop smoking for yourself, do it for your family and loved ones. You'll be protecting their health from the effects of your cigarette smoke and protecting them from the emotional trauma they would endure if you were to get cancer.

As if smoking weren't bad enough, people who smoke and drink are at even greater risk of cancer. People with these two habits experience a marked increase in the incidence of cancers of the esophagus, stomach and pancreas. Those at greatest risk drink and smoke *at the same time,* holding the alcohol and cigarette smoke in their mouths for a brief moment before swallowing. Research indicates when people smoke and drink at the same time, a mutagenic chemical called ethyl nitrite appears in their breath. This chemical is probably a powerful carcinogen; the chemical is not formed from smoking or drinking alone.

If you want to protect yourself from cancers of the esophagus, stomach and pancreas, stop smoking, and reduce the frequency and quantity of alcohol you drink to moderate levels. By moderate I mean 3 ounces of hard liquor or two 5-ounce glasses of wine or two 12-ounce glasses of beer a day, no more than 5 days a week. If you can't or won't stop these habits, at least don't smoke and drink at the same time.

DOES DIET CAUSE CANCER?

Results of several recent government-funded studies show a significant link between cancer and diet. As many as 45% of the cancer cases in this country may be due to diet. This evidence is hopeful news because we have more control over what food we put into our mouths than we do over what's in the air we breathe or the water we drink. It's not the preservatives, dyes or pesticides in our food that seem to matter— it's the *foods* we choose to eat that are significant in causing or preventing cancer.

The Committee on Diet and Nutrition, of the National Academy of Science, points the cancer-causing finger at fat intake and fiber intake. Studies indicate a high-fat diet increases the risk of developing breast, prostate and colon cancers. It appears we typically eat twice as much fat as is good for us. Approximately 40% of the calories in a typical diet come from fat in meat, milk, butter, cheese, sour cream, cooking oil, salad oil, margarine, fried foods, pastry, snack foods and ice cream.

The American Heart Association has been urging us to reduce our dietary fat to 30% of our caloric intake, but cancer researchers now believe a diet as low as 10 to 20% fat is needed to prevent cancer. Reducing dietary fat to 10% would be very difficult because the diet would seem unpalatable. However, a diet containing 20 to 25% fat can be tasty and offers protection from cancer when compared to our typical diet. The risk-reducing nutrition plan, page 186, is based on 20% fat, which helps protect you from cancer and heart disease.

A high-fat diet seems to affect the hormone levels in men and women, shifting hormone ratios and concentrations toward conditions favoring the development of cancer. A low-fat diet results in hormone levels that discourage cancer; breast and prostrate cancers are influenced by hormones.

Colon cancer is encouraged by a high-fat diet because to digest fat, your body produces bile acids. Many researchers believe bile acids encourage the growth of colon cancer. So the more fat you eat, the higher the concentration of bile acids in your colon. Cut down on fat, and you help lower your risk.

Diets that are high in fiber help reduce the risks of cancers of the breast and colon. The reason for the link is unclear, but the association is real. A high-fiber diet protects against these cancers, possibly because the fiber encourages frequent, bulky bowel movements that speed fat, bile acids and other carcinogenic agents through the bowels.

The type of fiber offering the most protection is *insoluble fiber*—cellulose, hemicellulose and lignin. Cellulose and hemicellulose are found in whole grains; lignin is found in whole grains, fruits and vegetables. *Soluble fiber,* which dissolves in water, is not protective against cancer. This type of fiber includes gums, mucilages and pectins; these are found primarily in fruits and vegetables.

The best source of insoluble fiber is bran contained in whole wheat; oat bran is also an excellent source of insoluble fiber. Eat whole grains every day. Half a cup of 100% whole-bran cereal has the same amount of fiber as three slices of whole-wheat bread. It's a good idea to start every day with a breakfast of 100% bran mixed with a more tasty cereal, such as Shredded Wheat, corn flakes or oatmeal.

A study carried out by Dr. Deborah Winn at the National Cancer Institute showed women who eat three or more servings of fruits or vegetables a day have *half* the amount of cancers of the throat and mouth as those who eat less than 1-1/2 servings a day. Another study revealed that women who ate a diet high in fiber and beta-carotene, which are found in fruits and vegetables, had lower rates of ovarian cancer. The same diet offers some protection to people who smoke cigarettes or who drink alcohol heavily, though it cannot reduce their cancer risk to the level of people who do not have these bad habits.

CHOOSE ANTI-CANCER FOODS

Scientists are reasonably confident beta-carotene and various retinoids (plant pigments that are precursors of vitamin A) are promising anti-cancer agents. Preliminary research shows these substances redirect cancerous cells back to their normal pathways of growth. Beta-carotene and retinoids seem to reduce the risk of lung, bladder, intestinal and larynx cancers, and possibly other cancers as well. At this time, no one knows the exact amount of either substance needed for protection; more research needs to be done.

You can purchase a tablet form of beta-carotene, but don't self-prescribe it. No one knows how much is the right amount, and too much vitamin A is highly toxic! The maximum dosage of vitamin A should be 5,000 to 10,000 units—20,000 units is likely to be toxic. There is no commercial product available for retinoids, even though they seem to have the most substantial evidence as a cancer-inhibiting agent. You can eat a well-balanced diet rich in vegetables containing beta-carotene and retinoids to provide much of the protection you need.

I recommend you eat one or two servings of dark-green, orange, deep-yellow or red fruits or vegetables every day. Deeply pigmented vegetables are rich in beta-carotene and retinoids. Good sources include carrots, red pepper, beets, spinach, broccoli, sweet potatoes, acorn squash, pumpkin, tomatoes, kale, collards, apricots, peaches, mangos, dates and prunes.

A large-scale experiment in which thousands of physicians are taking 30mg of beta-carotene every day for 5 years is being carried out at this time. Results will not be available until 1988. There's probably no harm in your taking 30mg of beta-carotene every other day, but whether or not this is the right amount, no one can yet say. Eating foods rich in beta-carotene will probably be more beneficial than a pill because you get fiber as well.

Vitamin C has been shown to have beneficial effects as a protective agent against cancer. Research sponsored by the National Cancer Institute indicates vitamin C enhances the immune system and stimulates the production of immune cells (T-lymphocytes) and interferon. This provides protection against certain cancers, particularly cancers of the stomach and esophagus. Vitamin C also inhibits nitrite and nitrate from combining with amines to form carcinogenic nitrosamines.

My advice is to *not* load up with large doses of vitamin C in the belief you are helping yourself. Too much vitamin C—more than 1 gram a day—may cause imbalances in other beneficial body substances, or it might be toxic. Excess vitamin C blocks the absorption of beta-carotene, which is a promising anti-cancer agent. It can also mobilize and diminish calcium from your bones and cause dozens of other harmful effects.

I recommend no more than 200 to 500mg of vitamin C a day in pill form. If you eat at least one food rich in vitamin C at every meal, you can easily reach 500mg with a diet that includes plenty of fruits and vegetables. Vitamin C is soluble in water and is destroyed by high heat and air. Use the freshest vegetables possible; cook them briefly in a small amount of water.

These foods give the amounts required to reach the RDA of vitamin C, which is 60mg:

1 small green pepper	1 grapefruit	6 ounces of grapefruit juice
1 cup of cauliflower	1 stalk of broccoli	1 orange
2 baked potatoes	1/2 cup of Brussels sprouts	4 ounces of orange juice

---

In addition, lemon, lime, strawberries and cantaloupe are all rich in vitamin C. Citrus juices are naturally high in vitamin C, but other fruit juices may be fortified with vitamin C and are also good sources. Each meal should contain one or more of these foods.

Scientists have found evidence that eating foods in the cabbage family, often called *cruciferous plants* after their Latin family name Cruciferae, may also provide protection against cancer. These foods contain a cancer-inhibiting substance—

dithiolthione—that is particularly effective against cancer of the colon. Though the evidence is not conclusive, it can't harm you to eat these vegetables once a day or at least three or four times a week. Vegetables to include in your diet are broccoli, cauliflower, cabbage, kale, kohlrobi, Brussels sprouts and watercress.

FOLLOW THE CANCER-PREVENTION DIET

If you are serious about following a diet to reduce your risk of cancer, it means changing your eating habits considerably from your average diet. But it doesn't mean your menus have to be boring. Include at least two servings of fruits and vegetables daily, with one serving from the high-vitamin-C group, two servings a day from the high-vitamin-A group and at least three or four servings a week of cruciferous vegetables.

Eat whole grains every day, substituting whole-wheat, whole-grain or oatmeal bread for white bread. Cut the amount of fat you eat by trimming meat carefully before cooking and avoiding butter sauces and rich desserts. Switch from whole milk to skim milk, and use low-fat cottage cheese instead of regular cottage cheese.

Eat red meat only once a week. Choose fish or skinless chicken at other meals. Eat a meatless dinner at least once a week, and rely on beans, grains and low-fat dairy products as your protein source.

It's important to eat a variety of foods. Fruits and grains keep your diet healthy and provide you with the maximum amount of vitamins and minerals you need.

Begin gradually to change your eating habits. Once you begin eating well, it will stay with you for the rest of your life.

There are some things to avoid as you begin to change your eating habits. Avoid frying or broiling meat. Reserve charcoal-grilled or smoked meats for special occasions because these methods of cooking can cause aromatic hydrocarbons, which are carcinogenic, to form in the meat. Avoid salt-cured or salt-pickled foods and those with sodium nitrate because they may contain nitrosamines.

CURES THAT DO NOT WORK

The National Academy of Sciences recommends eating foods rich in vitamin A and C, as well as eating cabbage-family vegetables. They do not advocate massive doses of selenium, zinc or vitamin E. Despite claims by popular self-proclaimed nutritionists, there is no evidence these substances offer any protection—in fact, they can be dangerous if overused.

Selenium is a trace mineral. It is a powerful anti-oxidant, as is beta-carotene, and it is important to your cells' metabolism. You receive selenium from fish, vegetables and meat, and it is unlikely you need additional sources because the body requires only small quantities.

Selenium is a metal, like lead and arsenic, so excess selenium in the body can be harmful and toxic. Your body does need it; standard vitamin-mineral preparations usually contain between 10 and 15mg of selenium. This is probably a safe level, but I would not advise a higher dose. It doesn't prevent cancer, and no matter what self-proclaimed experts say, megadoses are not safe.

Your body needs only tiny amounts of *zinc*. Any claims that it prevents or cures cancer are unfounded. Let me warn you that excess zinc from vitamin preparations is related to an *increased* incidence of cancer; too much zinc can also diminish selenium absorption. Studies show excess zinc can upset the balance of copper in your system, which can hasten development of hardening of the arteries. Some people's perception of zinc's benefits is another example of how pseudoscientists hoax people into throwing away their money and possibly damaging their health.

The benefits of *vitamin E* have also been heralded but without scientific proof. Vitamin E is fat soluble, and it is stored by your body. If you eat margarine and whole grains, you won't be deficient in vitamin E, and the probability of any benefit from additional amounts is doubtful. I do not recommend more than 400mg a day of vitamin E.

All dietary substances must be taken in proper proportion to each other. The risk of harm from taking megadoses of any vitamin or mineral far outweighs any potential benefits you might obtain.

You must understand cancer is not a single-pathway process, and no single agent will protect you. You must do many things to significantly lower your risk from cancer. It's safer to eat a good, healthy diet rich in fruits, vegetables and grains, and low in fats and meats than it is to swallow vitamin and mineral pills.

HOW DO YOU DETECT CANCER?

No one wants to get cancer, but detecting it early is one of the surest roads to a cure. A doctor's exam and certain laboratory tests can often detect cancer before any obvious symptoms appear. A family history of any type of cancer warrants careful scrutiny by your personal physician.

If you are a woman, examine your breasts every month, 1 week after your period ends. An internal examination and a breast exam by your gynecologist once a year, beginning when you are 20, is recommended. Pap tests should be done twice, 1 year apart, then every 3 years after age 20. Because cervical cancer is so slow to develop, this test is not needed more often unless you are at special risk. However, if you have genital herpes, a Pap test is recommended every 6 months. Don't overlook a yearly exam because you don't need a Pap smear. An exam is important to screen for cancers of the ovaries and other organs.

If you or your mother took DES, you should be examined more frequently, such as every 2 months. In older women, or women at special risk, regular mammograms are recommended, especially if there is suspicion of a breast mass. Your doctor may suggest one be done when you are 35 as a baseline for comparison if problems arise later. Discuss this with your physician.

Examine your skin regularly, and note any changes in pigment or size of existing moles or the appearance of new moles or sores that won't heal. Bring any changes to the immediate attention of your physician. Even innocuous-looking moles can have deadly potential.

Other conditions warrant special observation. There's a question as to the safety of regular chest X-rays, but I personally feel X-rays are the only possible means of detecting lung cancer while still curable. I recommend a chest X-ray every 6 months if you smoke. If you are a carrier of hepatitus-B virus, your physician should know about it; exams can be done to detect liver cancer. If you've had X-ray *treatment* during childhood, especially to the neck, your doctor should routinely screen you for thyroid cancer.

If you're over 50, have routine examinations of the colon by the scoping method or by X-ray, especially if you experience any unexplained change in your bowel routine or a bloody or black stool. Examination of the stool for microscopic blood should be done at least annually after age 40, and a digital rectal exam is recommended to screen for prostate and rectal tumors. These tests may detect cancer in its early stages when treatment provides a fairly high cure rate.

The greatest risk of contracting cancer seems to be from smoking cigarettes or using tobacco. Another risk is a high-fat diet lacking in fruits, vegetables and grain fiber. You can feel confident you're doing your best to prevent cancer from wrecking your life if you don't smoke and if you eat a healthy diet. Regular exercise provides further protection. Why not begin now?

9.

WHAT ARE YOUR RISKS OF DIABETES?

TAKE THIS TEST TO MEASURE YOUR
DIABETES RISK

This test measures your risk of developing Type-II diabetes. Circle the score for each characteristic that applies to you. Total the score, then check your risk category on page 110.

Weight

Choose any that apply.

You are:
+ 6   Overweight by 20%
+ 10   Overweight by 30% or more
+ 4   Overweight and have been since age 20 or before
+ 8   Overweight and eat a diet including refined sugars, such as cake, cookies, candy, soft drinks
+ 5   Overweight by 20% or more and do not exercise fairly vigorously for 30 minutes at least 3 times a week
+ 4   Overweight and the extra fat on your body is predominantly in your belly, if you are a man, or in your belly and above the waist (rather than just in your hips and thighs) if you are a woman

Diet

Choose any that apply.

+5   Eat cookies, cake, candy, sugared soft drinks or other sweets as dessert or snacks 3 or more times a day

+3   Eat cookies, cake, candy, sugared soft drinks or other sweets as dessert or snacks about twice a day

+2   Eat cookies, cake, candy, sugared soft drinks or other sweets as dessert or snacks about once a day

+1   Eat cookies, cake, candy, sugared soft drinks or other sweets as dessert or snacks several times a week

+1   Eat fatty cuts of steak, hamburger, pork and/or lamb 3 times a week

+2   Eat fatty cuts of steak, hamburger, pork and/or lamb 5 times a week

+3   Eat fatty cuts of steak, hamburger, pork and/or lamb more than 5 times a week

+1   Eat fatty processed meats, such as bologna, sausage or ham, twice a week

+2   Eat fatty processed meats, such as bologna, sausage or ham, 3 to 5 times a week

+3   Eat fatty processed meats, such as bologna, sausage or ham, more than 5 times a week

+1   Eat generous amounts of butter or margarine

+1   Eat fried foods several times a week

+2   Eat fried foods almost every day

+1   Eat rich desserts or ice cream several times a week

+2   Eat rich desserts or ice cream almost every day

+1   Eat cheese (except low-fat cottage cheese) several times a week

+2   Eat cheese (except low-fat cottage cheese) almost every day

+1   Eat empty-calorie foods or processed foods several times a week

+2   Eat empty-calorie foods or processed foods almost every day

−2   Eat at least 2 slices of whole-grain bread a day

−2   Eat a high-fiber cereal at least 3 times a week

−3   Eat cooked dried beans, such as navy or kidney beans, or lentils 3 or more times a week

−3   Eat at least 3 servings of high-fiber fruits or vegetables a day

Blood Sugar

Choose any that apply.

+ 10   You have recently been diagnosed as having hypoglycemia (low blood sugar)

+ 10   You have recently been diagnosed as having slightly elevated blood sugar

Family History

Choose any that apply.

+ 10   One or more grandparents with adult-onset diabetes

+ 12   One parent with adult-onset diabetes

+ 25   Both parents with adult-onset diabetes

+ 10   Brother or sister with adult-onset diabetes

+ 25   Identical twin with adult-onset diabetes

Personal

Choose any that apply.

+ 2   You are taking, or took, birth-control pills for 5 or more years

+ 2   You have been pregnant more than 5 times

+ 3   You are taking, or took, cortisone or cortisonelike medication for more than 6 months

+ 2   You are taking, or took, thiazide diuretics for 2 years or longer

+ 2   You are taking, or took, phenytoin (Dilantin and other brand names) for epilepsy or irregular heartbeat for 6 months or longer

INTERPRETING YOUR SCORE

To determine your score, add all scores from the categories. Check your total score below to see if your health and your life are at risk. You may be referred to the risk-reducing nutrition plan, page 186, or the risk-reducing exercise plan, page 226.

0 to 5   **Low Risk**—Your risk of developing diabetes is low. Your genetic history is in your favor, and your lifestyle habits give you extra protection.

6 to 20   **Moderate Risk**—You are at moderate risk of developing diabetes. If your family history is putting you at risk, follow the risk-reducing nutrition plan and the risk-reducing exercise plan to help protect yourself from developing the condition.

21 to 34 **High Risk**—You are at high risk of developing diabetes. Family history is one significant factor in this illness, but maintaining optimum weight and eating a diet rich in complex carbohydrates and low in fat and simple sugars will help lower your risk. Follow the risk-reducing nutrition plan and the risk-reducing exercise plan.

35 +   **Very High Risk**—You are at very high risk of developing diabetes. Your family history, coupled with your poor eating habits and overweight, are jeopardizing your health. Lose weight now, and follow the risk-reducing nutrition plan and the risk-reducing exercise plan to help lower your risks.

What Are Your Risks of Diabetes?

Diabetes is a serious disease. The popular notion that diabetes is merely a condition of elevated blood sugar fails to acknowledge that high blood sugar is only one manifestation of the disease. Few diseases have as much of an impact on *all* parts of the body as diabetes. In serious cases, diabetes impairs circulation and hardens arteries, resulting in kidney disease, gangrene of the legs and heart attacks. Tiny hemorrhages in the retina may cause blindness.

People with diabetes must constantly be alert for diabetic involvement of the kidneys, heart, liver, arterial system and nervous system. About 10 million Americans have diabetes; half of them don't even know it!

WHAT IS DIABETES?

The exact causes of diabetes are unknown. For some unknown reason, the pancreas in a person with diabetes does not manufacture enough insulin to "burn up" all the sugars and starches the person eats. Or if enough insulin is produced, it is somehow blocked from doing its job. Unmetabolized sugars and starches increase the sugar content of the blood and are passed through the kidneys into the urine.

Type-I, diabetes mellitus, (insulin-dependent diabetes) is the more severe form of diabetes. It may develop any time from infancy through old age, though it usually appears in childhood. For this reason it was previously called *juvenile diabetes.* Complications, especially of the kidneys, eyes and vascular system, frequently occur with Type-I diabetes. Insulin is required to control the disease—it cannot be controlled by diet or exercise alone.

Type-II, adult-onset diabetes mellitus (usually non-insulin-dependent diabetes) often appears during adult years, with no sign of diabetes prior to this. Its consequences can be as severe as those of Type-I, but it can usually be controlled by diet and exercise alone. Some cases of Type-II diabetes are more difficult to control because the patient refuses to follow dietary recommendations, and medication may be required. This form of diabetes develops in susceptible people due to lifelong habits of overeating. It is linked to obesity and overweight, along with a genetic predisposition for the condition.

Many doctors believe overweight and obesity actually cause Type-II diabetes. The pancreas and insulin action become overpowered by the excess food the body must cope with. About 80% of all people with Type-II diabetes are obese. In those over age 40, obese people suffer diabetes 5 times more often.

Even if you have a family history of Type-II diabetes, you don't have to contract the illness. The genetic aspect may be kept dormant if you follow a healthy diet, control your weight and exercise regularly. If you have a parent with Type-II diabetes, you are at risk, but you can reduce your risk of developing the disease. Maintain an ideal weight, eat a balanced diet and become physically active. You don't need to reduce carbohydrates if they are cereal grains, fruits and vegetables, but you must watch your intake of sweets, such as cakes and candies.

Although Type-II diabetes is controllable, if it develops and is ignored, the disease can damage the cardiovascular system as severely as Type-I diabetes. Doctors usually consider this type of diabetes less worrisome than Type-I *only* because it is easier to control once the condition is diagnosed.

In *some* people with Type-II diabetes, the disease does not interfere with their way of life, including their diet. Few complications occur, and they live a long life. Unfortunately, this is not the case for *most* people with Type-II diabetes. If insulin is required to control it, you may have vascular complications. But this warning is not limited only to those requiring insulin; if *any* type of diabetes gets out of control, consequences can be grim.

A common test for diabetes is the glucose-tolerance test. This test measures how much your blood sugar rises after you receive a test dose of glucose. If your blood sugar is elevated and does not return to normal within a specific period of time, this indicates there may be a possibility of diabetes.

This test is performed by taking a blood specimen after 3 days of normal eating (not avoiding carbohydrates, which makes test results abnormal), followed by an over-night fast. Blood samples are taken at the end of fasting, then at 1/2 hour, 1 hour, 2 hours, 3 hours and 4 hours after ingesting a carbohydrate load (75 grams of glucose) in a mixture given at the doctor's office or from a prescribed meal. If you're worried about hypoglycemia (low blood sugar), tests should also be done at 5 and 6 hours.

A simpler test is to take a blood sample at the end of fasting and another specimen 2 hours after drinking the glucose. If results are normal, this test rules out diabetes. You can also be tested for the effectiveness and quantity of the insulin your pancreas produces if you already have Type-II diabetes. If you're deficient in insulin quantity, you will require insulin supplement to control the disease.

DIABETES AS A RISK FACTOR FOR ATHEROSCLEROSIS

People who have either type of diabetes have an increased risk of atherosclerosis, and damage to their circulatory system can be serious. Unlike other causes of heart disease, diabetes causes the *smaller* vessels within the heart muscle to clog. These cannot be corrected with bypass surgery in the same way as clogging of larger coronary arteries.

Small blood vessels elsewhere in the body are also affected by diabetes. For instance, small vessels in the kidney may be injured by diabetes, resulting in progressive and chronic kidney failure. In older diabetics, leg vessels, particularly below the knee, can become so narrowed that inadequate blood supply reaches the feet, resulting in ulcers and possibly gangrene. Cataracts and damage to the eye's retina are other serious complications of diabetes.

When diabetes exists in conjunction with other risk factors for atherosclerosis, such as high blood pressure and high serum-cholesterol levels, your risk of heart disease is considerable.

CAN YOU AVOID DIABETES?

You have a higher risk of developing diabetes if you eat improperly and excessively, which may result in diminished insulin effectiveness. Being overweight is the *greatest* risk factor of developing Type-II diabetes, which is a risk factor of developing heart disease. Having the diabetic vascular condition predisposes you to atherosclerosis. When the two are present together, every organ in your body suffers greater risk of serious disease at an accelerated pace.

Even if you have a genetic predisposition toward diabetes, you may be able to avoid developing the disease. Your lifestyle—eating habits, exercise habits and weight— may trigger Type-II diabetes if you are susceptible to it. If you lead a healthy life, the disease may remain latent and never manifest itself.

Every time you eat sugars and starches, your pancreas secretes insulin. This enables carbohydrates to be metabolized, broken down and stored in the liver and muscles as glycogen. If your pancreas is challenged excessively over the years, insulin effectiveness becomes diminished. A larger amount of sugar remains unmetabolized in the bloodstream, indicating the beginning of diabetes. If you overwork your system with excess food, you may bring diabetes on yourself.

If Type-II diabetes is detected early, it is possible to overcome it. By reducing your caloric intake, limiting carbohydrates to nourishing complex carbohydrates, eliminating excess sugar and getting more exercise, you can prevent diabetes from becoming full-blown and doing serious damage.

Exercise is important in preventing and controlling diabetes because it burns up serum glucose. Exercise also helps you keep your weight under control. If you take insulin, it's important to exercise regularly and consistently because a change may affect the amount of insulin your body requires. A routine should be worked out very carefully with your doctor.

HOW TO LOWER YOUR RISK OF DIABETES

If you have developed diabetes because of lifelong, or even recent, overeating, it's possible that adopting healthy living habits can help reverse this condition.

A sound nutrition plan that offers a minimum of fat, is low in meat protein and high in complex carbohydrates will help reverse the condition and reduce the risk of complications. This means not overeating unnecessary simple carbohydrates, such as sugar, soft drinks, cake, ice cream and candy, while supplying the body with nourishing complex carbohydrates, such as grains, cereals and vegetables.

Recent research published in the *American Journal of Clinical Nutrition,* the *British Medical Journal* and the *Diabetes Journal* indicates dietary fiber may help control high blood sugar. Undigested fiber from a high-fiber diet absorbs sugar in the intestines, keeping the level of glucose in the bloodstream lower. A high-fiber diet is healthy for other reasons as well—it may help prevent certain forms of cancer and help overweight people lose weight.

Fiber helps diabetics control their blood-sugar level. A high-fiber diet may actually help prevent diabetes.

If you have diabetes or are at risk of developing it, the risk-reducing nutrition plan is essential to your good health. But you *must* understand you must follow the new diet for the rest of your life! If you revert to bad habits and challenge your insulin mechanism, your body will revert to the diabetic state, making it more difficult to control the condition.

Exercise is also very important in controlling diabetes and preventing its complications. Running, swimming, dancing, cross-country skiing, hiking, bicycling, racquetball and tennis (all aerobic exercises) help burn excess glucose and assist carbohydrate metabolism. The risk-reducing exercise program, page 226, will help you control diabetes if followed under your doctor's supervision.

The primary ways to avoid developing diabetes include maintaining normal weight, not overeating unnecessary sugars, supplying your body with nourishing carbohydrates and including regular physical activity in your daily routine. You can protect yourself to some extent from developing diabetes and its serious complications by eating right and getting more exercise!

10.

THE RISK FACTORS OF OSTEOPOROSIS

*TAKE THIS TEST TO MEASURE YOUR
OSTEOPOROSIS RISK*

This test measures your risk of osteoporosis. Circle the score for each characteristic that applies to you. Total the score, then check your risk category on page 117.

Diet

Choose any that apply.
+ 10   Consumed less than 1 quart of milk a day, or the equivalent, in adolescence
+ 10   Consumed less than 1 quart of milk a day, or the equivalent, in your 20s and 30s
+ 10   Consumed less than 1 quart of milk a day, or the equivalent, in your 40s
+ 15   Consumed less than 1 quart of milk a day, or the equivalent, after 50
 +5   Drink more than two cups of coffee a day
 +5   Drink more than two soft drinks a day
+ 10   Drink more than two 5-ounce glasses of wine or two 12-ounce glasses of beer or 3 ounces of alcohol 5 times a week
 +5   Frequently use antacids containing aluminum

Family History

Choose any that apply.

+10 Female
−30 Male
+10 Caucasian of Northern European ancestry
−40 Caucasian of Southern European or Mediterranean ancestry
+10 Oriental or Asian ancestry
−60 Black or African ancestry
 +5 Fair skin
 +5 Thin or wrinkled skin
 +5 Red or blond hair
+10 Small bones
 +5 Small muscles
 +5 Have always been underweight
+10 Blood relative who had osteoporosis—lost height, developed dowager's hump or broke a hip

Health

Choose any that apply.

+10 Currently smoke 1 pack of cigarettes a day
+15 Currently smoke 2 packs of cigarettes a day
+10 Previously smoked cigarettes—more than 10 years
 +5 Previously smoked cigarettes—less than 10 years
 -30 Estrogen-replacement therapy from menopause on
 +5 Early menopause or surgical removal of ovaries after 45
+10 Early menopause or surgical removal of ovaries before 45
+10 Periodontal gum disease
+10 Diabetes requiring insulin control
+20 Long-term cortisone or steroid use
 -15 Overweight

Exercise

Choose any that apply.

+15 Sedentary lifestyle during 20s
+10 Sedentary lifestyle during 30s
+10 Sedentary lifestyle during 40s
+15 Sedentary lifestyle during 50s
+15 Sedentary lifestyle in 60s and beyond

INTERPRETING YOUR SCORE

To determine your score, add all scores from the categories. Check your total score below to see if your health and your life are at risk. You may be referred to the risk-reducing nutrition plan, page 186, or the risk-reducing exercise plan, page 226.

0 to 65   **Low Risk**—You are at low risk of developing osteoporosis. If you scored points due to heredity, you are taking proper care of yourself, and that's why your risk is low. Continue good health habits to maintain your low risk of the disease.

70 to 130   **Moderate Risk**—You are at moderate risk of developing osteoporosis. There's little you can do to change your genetic endowment, but changing lifestyle habits that increased your score will help lower your risk. Follow the risk-reducing nutrition plan and the risk-reducing exercise plan.

135 to 195   **High Risk**—You are at high risk of developing osteoporosis. Eat a calcium-rich diet, follow the risk-reducing nutrition plan and follow the risk-reducing exercise program to lower your risk.

200+   **Very High Risk**—Your family background and your living habits conspire against you. It may not be too late to prevent further bone loss, but increasing your bone mass may not be possible. Diet, exercise and possibly estrogen replacement are your best keys to reversing or slowing the condition. Follow the risk-reducing nutrition plan and the risk-reducing exercise plan. Don't wait; the time to start is now!

117

The Risk Factors of Osteoporosis

We all probably know an elderly person who fell and broke a hip. Did you know it's probable the hip broke *before* the fall? The fractured bone caused the fall, not the other way around! Deteriorating bones can become so thin and weak that the pressure exerted on them simply by supporting body weight while walking can be enough to cause a fracture.

Many older people fear such an accident because it often leads to a dramatic decline in health and mobility. The fracture may never heal properly, and surgical implantation of a metal pin may be required. The bed rest and inactivity necessary during healing of the hip can lead to other problems, such as depression.

The National Institute of Health reports that among the 200,000 hip fractures suffered by older people in this country every year, 160,000 are related to a disease called *osteoporosis*. Nearly 32,000 people die from complications of the fracture, such as development of pneumonia or pulmonary embolism.

Osteoporosis is a condition in which the bones become thin and weak. It often occurs with age and has many manifestations—a broken hip is just one. The first indication of osteoporosis is often gradual loss of height over the years. Sometimes a dramatic loss of height occurs—from 3 to 8 inches in a few years. This is a result of weakened bones in the spine becoming porous and brittle and compressing like stacked Shredded-Wheat biscuits, from no more stress than that imposed by walking or carrying out ordinary daily activities. As the vertebrae crush, the spine bends forward, resulting in the *dowager's hump*.

Broken wrists are also common. When you fall, you naturally try to protect yourself by stretching out your arms. If the force of the fall is great enough—or the bones weak enough—you sustain a broken bone, often a broken wrist. Wrist fractures are most common in older women.

Bone weakening doesn't have to be an inevitable part of old age, as many people fear. Osteoporosis, like heart disease, cancer and diabetes, is often a disease of lifestyle. Some people are at greater risk than others because of genetic endowment. However, most can and should take positive steps to avoid this debilitating, disfiguring disease through good nutrition and regular exercise. The time to start is while you're young!

Strong bones formed and maintained during youth and middle age are important in keeping you strong and vigorous during later years. It's difficult, if not impossible, to make bones that were weak during youth and middle age stronger and denser once osteoporosis begins. Osteoporosis may start slowly and insidiously as early as age 35 in women but much later in men.

According to the Surgeon General, as many as 15 million Americans have osteoporosis; each year 6 million of them suffer broken bones as a result of the disease. Among women, 25% of all women over 65 have osteoporosis, and among men over 65, 12.5% of them suffer from this bone-weakening disease.

Bones have a dense, hard outer shell and a honeycombed interior filled with marrow; a network of blood vessels traverses the bones. Vessels deliver the nutrients and oxygen a bone needs for good health and take away the newly manufactured red and white blood cells made by the bone marrow. Bone is always in a dynamic state of change. Old bone tissue is broken down and new bone laid down in a continual exchange system regulated by hormones and the concentration of bone-building materials in the blood.

Bone is made of minerals laid over a framework of collagen protein—this combination makes them strong. Calcium and phosphate are present in quantity along with small amounts of fluorine, magnesium and zinc. Trace amounts of copper, potassium, sodium, iodine, chromium, sulfur, manganese and molybdenum also make up bone tissue. Bone acts as a storehouse for all these minerals—99% of your body's calcium is in your bones and teeth. When your body's tissues, organs and muscles lack minerals, bone is dissolved to free them.

The thyroid gland produces the hormone calcitonin, which helps conserve bone calcium. The parathyroid gland produces the hormone parathormone, which regulates blood calcium levels. Muscles and nerves need a specific level of calcium in the blood to function properly. These two hormones act together to keep the blood's calcium concentration at the proper concentration.

The adrenal glands also produce sex hormones needed for bone growth. Glucocorticoids encourage bone dissolution, while calcitonin encourages bone preservation. The sex hormones—estrogen in women and testosterone in men—also preserve bone. As these hormones decline with age, so does bone mass.

Normally, the constant flux of minerals in and out of the bones makes no consequence to bone health because bones are designed to be storehouses as well as supporting structures. But if your diet is deficient in calcium or your intestines are unable to absorb sufficient calcium, your parathyroid gland will send a chemical messenger to the bone and activate osteoclast activity. Calcium will be released into the bloodstream to maintain the necessary concentration in the blood. Chronic calcium deficiency leads to more bone being lost than is replaced—weakened, brittle bones result.

A vitamin-D deficiency can also result in osteoporosis because this vitamin plays an important role in calcium absorption. Without sufficient vitamin D, your intestines cannot absorb calcium from food. Vitamin D is found in certain foods, such as liver, tuna, cod liver oil, egg yolk, salmon and fortified milk. Your skin can also manufacture it from sunshine—15 to 60 minutes a day of sunshine is sufficient. A balanced diet or outdoor exercise provides adequate vitamin D.

DOES GENETIC PREDISPOSITION AFFECT OSTEOPOROSIS?

Men and women lose bone density as they age, but women suffer from the disease twice as frequently as men. Women's bones are usually 30% less dense. Hormones that keep bones dense drop off dramatically during menopause. Hormonal decline is more gradual in men,· so the disease develops later in life.

People of oriental ancestry are at greater risk than blacks or dark-complexioned people from Spain, Italy, Greece or the Middle East because their bones are not as large or as dense. Heredity plays an important primary role in the development of osteoporosis because it influences bone density and hormonal actions.

Blacks lose bone mass with age, but the progression is much slower than with whites. Loss of bone mass in blacks rarely progresses fast enough to result in fractured bones. If severe osteoporosis develops, it is usually the result of some other disease.

If you are petite or small-boned, you're at greater risk because your bones are smaller to begin with. Other characteristics exhibited by people susceptible to osteoporosis include flexible, loose joints; fallen arches; scoliosis; thin, loose skin that bruises easily; fair complexion; blond or red hair; freckled skin; periodontal disease.

You are at highest genetic risk of osteoporosis if you are a woman whose mother suffered from osteoporosis. But if your physical characteristics put you at risk and any of your close relatives—aunts, uncles and grandparents—had the disease, consider yourself at high risk.

NUTRITION CAN AFFECT YOUR RISK OF OSTEOPOROSIS

Good nutrition builds strong bones. Although bones are built from many minerals, insufficient dietary calcium seems to play a crucial role in the development of osteoporosis. Some authorities believe even a 50mg daily deficit over the course of 20 years can lead to brittle bones. As you age, your body absorbs less calcium from your intestines, so contrary to popular opinion, many adults need to eat as much *or more* calcium as growing children. Milk and milk products are the best sources of calcium.

Recently the National Institute of Health revised the recommended daily allowance of calcium. Previously, it was suggested adults needed 800mg of calcium a day. The panel of experts now strongly urges Americans get the following calcium levels:

- Adolescents: 1,500mg
- Pregnant and lactating women: 2,000mg
- Pregnant and lactating adolescents: 2,500mg
- Post-menopausal women: 1,500mg
- Women over 35: 1,000mg
- Older men: 1,000mg

If you have not been getting this much calcium, you are probably calcium deficient, and your bones are suffering. Milk and dairy products are the best sources of calcium, and skim or low-fat products are your healthiest choices—so study the following table to check out your calcium intake.

- Adolescents: 5 cups of skim milk/day
- Pregnant and lactating women: 6-1/2 cups of skim milk/day
- Pregnant and lactating women: 8-1/4 cups of skim milk/day
- Post-menopausal women: 5 cups of skim milk/day
- Women over 35: 3-1/3 cups of skim milk/day
- Older men: 3-1/3 cups of skim milk/day

Different kinds of milk contain different amounts of calcium. See the chart below. Differences may seem minimal, but if you count calcium, it may make a significant difference in the long-run to your calcium intake.

Type of Food	Amount of Calcium in 1 cup
• Whole milk	288mg
• Low-fat milk, 2% fat	297mg
• Low-fat milk, 2% fat, with non-fat milk solids	313mg
• Low-fat milk, 2% fat, protein-fortified	352mg
• Low-fat milk, 1% fat	300mg
• Low-fat milk, 1% fat, with non-fat dry milk added	313mg
• Low-fat milk, 1% fat, protein-fortified	349mg
• Skim milk	302mg
• Skim milk, with non-fat dry milk added	316mg
• Skim milk, protein-fortified	352mg
• Skim milk, dry instant	297mg
• Buttermilk, cultured, 1% fat	285mg
• Low-fat yogurt, 1% fat, with non-fat milk solids	326mg
• Low-fat yogurt, 1% fat, with non-fat milk solids, fruit-flavored	306mg
• Skim yogurt, with non-fat milk solids	355mg
• Calcium-fortified milk, 1% fat	500mg

HOW EXERCISE AFFECTS YOUR RISKS

Exercise builds strong bones; regular exercise that places weight on the bones is the only natural means of actually increasing bone mass. If you are sedentary at home and at work, you're placing yourself at higher risk of osteoporosis. It is unclear why this occurs, but exercise may stimulate hormonal changes that tell the bone to slow the breakdown and increase formation. Exercise also increases blood circulation, which is necessary to carry calcium, other minerals and hormones throughout the bones.

The dominant arm of a tennis player may be 15% denser and thicker than his other arm. Marathon runners have denser leg bones (the femur tibia) than non-athletes. Ballet dancers have large, strong, leg bones. It is a common observation that people confined to bed lose bone mass. Immobilized bones of paralyzed people become osteoporotic due to rapid calcium loss in the same way as bones confined to a cast for a long time.

The early astronauts of the Gemini missions lost total calcium and bone strength because of weightlessness, which puts no stress on the bones. Later Gemini astronauts were given a special exercise program to counteract this effect.

Many research studies support the observation that exercise increases bone mass. An important study carried out on women in their 80s by the University of Wisconsin showed those who exercised 30 minutes a day 3 times a week increased their total body calcium and bone density compared to women who did not exercise. Other studies showed a daily hour-long walk was effective in encouraging stronger bones.

HOW SMOKING, ALCOHOL AND MEDICATION AFFECT YOUR RISK

You're probably tired of hearing about all the bad things cigarette smoking does to your health, but here's another to add to the list. Smoking increases your risk of osteoporosis. No one knows exactly why this is, but the evidence is clear. Smoking may indirectly influence osteoporosis because women who are heavy smokers experience menopause on the average of 5 years earlier than non-smoking women.

Smokers also have impaired blood circulation, and this may mean calcium doesn't get to the bones as efficiently as it should. The chemical effects of nicotine and the slightly raised acidity of the blood in smokers may affect calcium metabolism.

Research published in the *Journal of Clinical Nutrition* showed women *and* men who had several drinks a day developed osteoporosis more readily than non-drinking people of similar background. This is because alcohol damages the liver and slows absorption of calcium in the intestines. The liver and kidneys change vitamin D to an active form needed for calcium absorption. Research also shows women who are heavy coffee or cola drinkers are more prone to osteoporosis.

Some medications can seriously interfere with the health of your bones. Long-term use of cortisone or similar steroid drugs for illnesses, such as rheumatoid-arthritis, asthma and lupus, encourages severe osteoporosis. Spine and rib fractures commonly occur among these steroid users because the drug increases bone loss and decreases new-bone formation. People with certain diseases of the thyroid or those under extreme stress produce excessive amounts of natural cortisonelike hormones; these also speed osteoporosis.

Diabetics requiring insulin are at risk of osteoporosis. Bone is usually lost after beginning insulin treatment or increasing insulin dosage. Diabetics usually have a 10% lower bone mass than similar non-diabetic people. Glucocosteroid hormones produced by the adrenal glands influence blood-sugar levels and calcium metabolism, which may explain the link between diabetes and osteoporosis.

Antacids containing aluminum indirectly interfere with calcium metabolism because the aluminum binds with phosphorous. This results in a phosphorous deficiency in the blood, which is replaced with phosphorous from the bones. Calcium is removed from the bones, along with the phosphorous, and excreted in the urine.

DIAGNOSING OSTEOPOROSIS

Diagnosing osteoporosis before symptoms, such as fractures, humped back or loss of height, are observable is difficult if not impossible. Osteoporosis cannot be detected by X-ray until the bones lose 30 to 40% of their calcium; by then the disease has progressed dangerously far. If you have suffered a fracture, an experienced doctor will be able to tell from the type and placement of the break if it resulted from osteoporosis.

Blood tests for calcium level reveal nothing about the state of your bones because calcium dissolves from your bones to maintain a constant level in the bloodstream. A series of urine tests may reveal too much calcium being lost from your body, but the results must be interpreted according to your health, diet and degree of exercise.

Researchers use a variety of methods to detect early osteoporosis, such as photon absorptionometry, CAT scan, isotopic bone scan and radiographic absorptionometry, which are not available to the general public. A chain of diagnostic centers that uses single-beam densiometers to measure the bone density of the wrists recently opened nationwide. This technique is controversial; many physicians feel the density of the wrist is not indicative of the density of the spine.

A technique called *dual photon absorptionometry* is becoming more widely available; this test can scan vertebrae, which is translucent bone. Although the diagnostic test is expensive, a woman at risk of osteoporosis may wish to be evaluated at menopause to help her and her doctor decide whether to use estrogen-replacement therapy.

Diagnosis of osteoporosis is really based more on evaluating risk factors and making physical observations. We all lose bone mass as we age, so it's important to take preventive measures. If you are at special risk, these measures are even more important in assuring your good health.

YOU CAN LOWER YOUR RISK OF OSTEOPOROSIS

There's nothing you can do to change your genetic risk of osteoporosis. But you can take preventive steps to dramatically inhibit your genetic destiny from coming to fruition.

The National Institute of Health recently advocated a significant increase in the daily recommended amount of calcium. The former recommendation was 800mg for adults of all ages; experts now recommend an increase to between 1,000 and 1,500mg per day, depending on sex and age. It is clear why osteoporosis is so widespread. Studies show the average American women gets only 450mg a day—an amount far below what is needed to sustain healthy bones.

Calcium is present in large quantities in milk and dairy products. Milk products also contain lactose, a sugar that increases calcium absorption from the bowel. Dairy products are the best sources of calcium in your diet and should be included in every meal. Milk is high in fat, so I recommend only skim or low-fat dairy products in the risk-reducing nutrition plan.

Many dark-green vegetables are high in calcium, but spinach, broccoli, collards and turnip greens contain oxalate crystals, which discourage calcium absorption. Include these foods in your diet, but don't consider them a good source of calcium.

Excessive phosphates in your diet may prevent or reduce calcium absorption. Phosphates are important components of bone, but they are not needed in the diet in the same way as calcium. Phosphates are found in red meat and in many food additives. The worst offenders, when it comes to overdoing phosphates, are soft drinks. I recommend you limit soft drinks to an occasional treat.

The risk-reducing nutrition plan provides three servings of dairy products a day. This is about 900mg or of three glasses of skim milk. Milk is also a high-protein food; my nutrition plan, page 186, provides small but adequate amounts of protein.

If you need more calcium than you can get from your food, I recommend you take calcium supplements to fulfill your calcium needs. It isn't practical for post-menopausal women (who may need fewer calories than more-active younger women) to drink five 8-ounce glasses of skim milk a day—the amount they would need to meet their calcium needs.

There are many kinds of calcium supplements available at the drugstore. The choice is complicated because many labels seem to be designed to conceal how many pills you'll need to take to get the necessary amount of calcium. I recommend you take *calcium carbonate* because this compound is easily absorbed, and more calcium is available in each pill than with many other compounds. Calcium compounds are large molecules with only a small percentage of calcium. Calcium carbonate is 40% calcium; a 500mg pill contains 200mg of calcium.

Calcium carbonate is the active ingredient in many antacids. A 500mg Tums, for example, contains 200mg of calcium. You may take Tums or a similar antacid as a calcium source as long as it doesn't contain sodium or aluminum. But you are also ingesting other unnecessary additives designed to make the tablet chewable.

Calcium phosphate does not dissolve well in the intestines, and only 29% of each pill is calcium. Too much phosphate can interfere with calcium absorption. Calcium gluconate pills are only 9% calcium, and calcium lactate are 13% calcium. A 600mg pill of calcium lactate contains only 78mg of calcium—to get 1,000mg of calcium, you'd need to take 13 pills! Calcium gluconate and calcium lactate are easily dissolved and absorbed, but calcium gluconate may irritate your stomach.

If you have reduced stomach acidity, take the calcium carbonate pills with a glass of water on an empty stomach because pills need to dissolve in your stomach acid. (Food dilutes the acid further.) Don't take them with a glass of milk because milk neutralizes stomach acids. If you're taking several tablets, try to take them throughout the day rather than all at once.

Ask your doctor's advice about taking calcium supplements. Supplements may increase the risk of kidney stones in susceptible people, especially those who drink small amounts of fluid. Your doctor can best advise you if you are at risk of developing kidney stones.

Do not take "natural" sources of calcium, such as dolomite. These may be contaminated with harmful levels of lead or arsenic. Several poisonings from these calcium supplements have been reported in medical literature.

DIET, EXERCISE AND HORMONES CAN HAVE AN EFFECT

A high-fiber diet may interfere with calcium absorption, but research on this point is contradictory. The high-fiber in the risk-reducing nutrition plan is not excessive and is necessary to protect you from other diseases, so don't be concerned. As long as your diet is rich in calcium and you take additional calcium supplements if you're post-menopausal, you'll get enough calcium.

High-protein diets may speed osteoporosis because calcium is lost from the bones to help metabolize excess protein. If you eat a high-protein diet, you lose needed calcium in your urine and feces. Red meat also contains phosphates, which may interfere with calcium absorption. My nutrition plan is not high in protein, a benefit that helps protect you from osteoporosis.

An added benefit of a calcium-rich diet is the protection it offers against developing high blood pressure. Many researchers believe a high-sodium, low-calcium diet may be a risk factor of developing high blood pressure. By getting plenty of calcium, you may help lower your risk of high blood pressure.

Exercise is also important. Getting enough exercise of the type that puts weight on your bones is essential in keeping your bones strong as you age. Even if you have dense bones to begin with and eat a calcium-rich diet, exercise keeps bones from deteriorating. It may be the only way to increase bone density if your bones have already become brittle.

Any kind of exercise involving movement that puts weight on your limbs helps prevent osteoporosis if it is done regularly. The exercise doesn't have to be strenuous—the constant movement is important. Good exercises include walking, running, hiking, jumping rope, skiing, swimming, bicycling, most competitive sports and even house and yard work, as long as you keep moving. The minimum amount of exercise is 1/2 hour a day at least 3 times a week. Your risk will be lower if you exercise for longer periods—up to 1 hour—every day.

The risk-reducing exercise plan, beginning on page 226, is designed to protect you from many diseases, including osteoporosis. If you follow it, you'll be protecting your heart and immune system, as well as your bones.

It has long been suspected that estrogen-replacement therapy begun during menopause prevents osteoporosis. When the ovaries age or are removed, the body is deprived of estrogen. Women who experience an early menopause around age 40 or a surgical menopause from having their ovaries and uterus removed have a higher risk of developing osteoporosis. Women athletes who train so hard that they stop having menstrual periods also show loss of bone calcium, even though they exercised. Once their periods return, bone loss stops. Overweight women have a lower risk of osteoporosis than normal-weight women—this is probably due to the extra estrogen produced in fatty tissue and the weight-bearing effect that overweight places on the bones.

Research designed to tell if aging or estrogen deficiency played a more important role in osteoporosis was done at the Mayo Clinic. It revealed the degree of osteoporosis in older women hinges more on the number of years the woman is past menopause than on her age. Lack of estrogen was most apparent in the years between 50 and 70.

Until recently, research did not prove estrogen replacement actually helped keep bones from becoming brittle. But a study done in Scotland followed women for 9 years. Of those women who took estrogen, 4% lost height, while 38% of those who did not take the drug lost height.

A British study of 1,000 women who took estrogen for 14 years showed wrist fractures among them were 70% below what would have been expected. Studies from the University of Washington and Yale University, which investigated risk factors of women who suffered hip and wrist fractures, revealed few fracture victims had taken estrogen. In 1983, the American Medical Association concluded estrogen prevents osteoporosis.

Estrogen slows calcium loss from the bones but does not stimulate new bone growth. It is important that estrogen replacement therapy be begun at the onset of menopause, *before* significant bone loss begins. You need to take estrogen for many years because stopping the hormone therapy may instigate rapid bone loss. The lowest dosage of estrogen needed to prevent osteoporosis is about 0.625mg, much less than the 2.5mg often needed to prevent hot flashes.

Estrogen-replacement therapy increases your risk of endometrial cancer (cancer of the lining of the uterus) from 2 to 20%. But this cancer is easy to detect and is slow spreading. Most medical researchers believe that combining estrogen replacement with progesterone reduces the increased risk of endometrial cancer.

A more serious risk from taking estrogen is development of heart disease, although this is controversial. Research done several years ago in Britain indicated that women who took estrogen had a 68% lower rate of heart attacks than women who did not. This protective effect may be due to selecting healthier women to begin with for estrogen treatment. A recent report from the Framingham project indicated women who take estrogen have a *greater* chance of developing heart disease than women who do not.

You must weigh many factors in deciding whether to take estrogen-replacement therapy. Are you at risk of osteoporosis? Are you at risk of cancer? Are you at risk of heart disease? If your first answer is yes but your other answers are no, estrogen replacement is probably advisable. If *all* your answers are yes, discuss the matter with your physician, who can help you weigh the risks of estrogen replacement against the benefits.

Studies show women commonly begin to lose bone mass at about age 35—some as early as age 25. About 20% of all women begin to lose bone mass rapidly beginning at menopause. If your bones are dense and strong, they contain more calcium and will remain strong, even as hormonal changes encourage calcium loss.

By eating a high-calcium diet and exercising about 1/2 hour a day, you'll considerably lower your risk of osteoporosis. But the time to start is not when you first notice you aren't as tall as you used to be or your shoulders are stooped and rounded. The time to start is now!

A lifetime adherence to the risk-reducing nutrition plan and the risk-reducing exercise plan, and estrogen replacement, if indicated, are your best chances for a lifetime of healthy, strong bones.

11.

THE RISK FACTORS OF STRESS

TAKE THIS TEST TO MEASURE YOUR
STRESS LEVEL

How you react to stress is more important to your health than the amount of stress you experience. This test measures the amount of stress you are under. Circle the score for each characteristic that applies to you. Total the score, then check your risk category on page 135.

Your Feelings About Yourself

Circle the number for each statement that reflects your feelings.
Column 1 = Always
Column 2 = Frequently
Column 3 = Occasionally
Column 4 = Rarely
Column 5 = Never

	COLUMNS				
	1	**2**	**3**	**4**	**5**
You feel in control of your life.	0	1	3	4	5
You are happy with your family and home life.	0	1	3	4	5
You like your work or your occupation.	0	1	3	4	5

	COLUMNS				
	1	**2**	**3**	**4**	**5**
You are proud of yourself or your achievements.	0	1	3	4	5
You are satisfied with your level of income.	0	1	3	4	5
You are satisfied with your friends.	0	1	3	4	5
You are often angry with the world around you.	15	14	5	1	0
You feel overwhelmed by your problems.	5	4	3	1	0
You see little chance to get ahead.	5	4	3	1	0
You feel as if no one appreciates your efforts.	5	4	3	1	0
You are depressed.	15	14	5	1	0
You are concerned about your health.	5	4	3	1	0

Your Behavior Patterns

Circle the number for each statement that reflects your feelings.
Column 1 = Always
Column 2 = Frequently
Column 3 = Occasionally
Column 4 = Rarely
Column 5 = Never

	1	**2**	**3**	**4**	**5**
You have an intense desire to get ahead.	6	5	3	0	0
You feel a constant desire to succeed.	6	5	3	0	0
You are easily irritated, annoyed or frustrated.	8	6	3	0	0
You get angry or feel hostile if you lose.	15	14	8	0	0
You feel angry or hostile toward your spouse.	20	18	10	1	0
You are competitive and must win in all situations.	7	6	3	1	0
You have many projects going at one time.	6	5	2	0	0
You are constantly bothered by incomplete work.	8	7	5	0	0
You laugh often and have a "good time."	0	0	5	14	15
You do many things yourself because it's easier to do it yourself or no one else is capable of doing it.	6	5	3	1	0
You plan ahead to leave time for relaxation and exercise.	0	0	2	4	5
You eat rapidly and don't sit and talk or enjoy your food.	4	3	2	0	0
You have headaches.	5	4	3	1	0

	COLUMNS				
	1	**2**	**3**	**4**	**5**
You have insomnia.	5	4	3	1	0
You feel bloated or have indigestion, constipation or diarrhea.	5	4	3	1	0
You lack interest in sex.	5	4	3	1	0

Events in Your Life

Circle the number for each statement that reflects your situation.
Column 1 = 6 months ago
Column 2 = 1 year ago
Column 3 = 1-1/2 years ago
Column 4 = 2 years ago
Column 5 = 3 years ago

	1	**2**	**3**	**4**	**5**
You moved out of state.	10	5	4	2	0
You moved to a new community in the same state.	8	4	3	1	0
You moved to a new residence in the same community.	5	4	3	1	0
Your community suffered a serious natural disaster.	15	10	8	5	0
Your home was destroyed in a natural disaster.	20	15	10	6	0
You suffered serious property damage but not complete destruction in a natural disaster.	15	10	8	5	0

Your Family

Circle the number for each statement that reflects your situation.
Column 1 = 6 months ago
Column 2 = 1 year ago
Column 3 = 1-1/2 years ago
Column 4 = 2 years ago
Column 5 = 3 years ago

	1	**2**	**3**	**4**	**5**
Your spouse died.	25	20	15	10	8
Your child died.	25	20	15	10	8
A relative to whom you were close died.	20	15	10	5	0

	COLUMNS				
	1	**2**	**3**	**4**	**5**
A close friend died.	20	15	10	5	0
You were divorced or separated.	20	15	10	5	0
You got married.	10	5	3	0	0
Your first child was born.	15	15	15	10	5
Another child was born.	10	10	10	10	10
You suffered a serious illness.	15	10	5	0	0
Your spouse suffered a serious illness.	15	10	5	0	0
Your child suffered a serious illness.	15	10	5	0	0
You have a parent or in-law who moved in with you and your family.	10	8	5	3	3
Your child has left home for college, work or marriage.	8	5	3	0	0
You were in trouble with the law.	8	5	3	0	0
Your spouse or child was in trouble with the law.	8	5	3	0	0

Your Family

Circle the number for each statement that reflects your situation.

Column 1 = Always
Column 2 = Frequently
Column 3 = Occasionally
Column 4 = Rarely
Column 5 = Never

	1	**2**	**3**	**4**	**5**
Your spouse drinks too much.	8	5	4	1	0
Your teenage children cause you serious concern.	10	8	5	1	0
You are responsible for caring for an ailing parent or in-law.	15	10	5	1	0
You and your spouse have heated arguments.	10	8	4	1	0
You feel close to your family and feel they would give you emotional or financial support if you needed it.	0	1	3	6	12

Your Employment or Occupation

Circle the number for each statement that reflects your situation.
Column 1 = 6 months ago
Column 2 = 1 year ago
Column 3 = 1-1/2 years ago
Column 4 = 2 years ago
Column 5 = 3 years ago

	COLUMNS				
	1	**2**	**3**	**4**	**5**
You were fired but are now employed.	15	10	6	1	0
You were fired and are still out of work.	20	15	15	10	10
You were laid off but are now employed.	12	8	6	0	0
You were laid off and are still out of work.	12	10	10	10	1
You have the same job but have a new boss.	8	6	1	0	0
You changed professions.	10	8	6	0	0
You changed jobs within the same profession.	6	4	2	0	0
You were promoted to a position with increased responsibility.	8	6	1	0	0
You were demoted to a position with less responsibility.	9	6	3	0	0
You retired.	10	8	6	5	3
Your spouse retired.	8	6	4	2	1
Your work hours changed.	2	1	0	0	0
You were given a lower raise than you expected.	5	2	1	0	0

Your Employment or Occupation

Circle the number for each statement that reflects your situation.
Column 1 = Always
Column 2 = Frequently
Column 3 = Occasionally
Column 4 = Rarely
Column 5 = Never

	1	2	3	4	5
You are seriously concerned about losing your job or your spouse losing his or her job.	8	6	4	1	0

	COLUMNS				
	1	2	3	4	5
You commute by car in heavy traffic.	6	5	4	1	0
You commute by public transportation in crowded or noisy conditions.	10	8	6	2	0
You commute to work by car or public transportation, 1/2 hour each way.	4	3	2	1	0
You commute to work by car or public transportation, 1 hour each way.	6	5	4	2	0
You commute to work by car or public transportation more than 1 hour each way.	8	6	4	2	0
You make out-of-town business trips.	10	8	4	1	0
You work under noisy conditions.	6	5	4	1	0
You get along well with your boss.	0	1	3	5	7
You get along well with your colleagues.	0	2	5	7	9
You do several projects at once.	7	5	3	0	0
You have rigid deadlines that are difficult to meet.	7	5	3	0	0
Your job or occupation is frustrating and brings little satisfaction or recognition.	9	6	3	2	0
You work overtime or long hours.	7	5	3	0	0
Your boss praises your work.	0	0	2	5	7
You have free time for fun, recreation or vacations.	0	0	2	5	7

Your Lifestyle

Circle the number for each statement that reflects your situation.
Column 1 = 6 months ago
Column 2 = 1 year ago
Column 3 = 1-1/2 years ago
Column 4 = 2 years ago
Column 5 = 3 years ago

	1	2	3	4	5
The number of family get-togethers you attend has changed.	3	2	1	0	0
The number of social events you attend has changed.	3	2	1	0	0

	COLUMNS				
	1	2	3	4	5
The number of vacations you take has changed.	3	2	1	0	0
You have lost friends.	5	4	3	0	0
You have made new friends.	5	4	3	0	0
Your sleeping habits have changed.	3	2	1	0	0
Your eating habits have changed.	3	2	1	0	0
Your drinking habits have changed.	3	2	1	0	0
Your smoking habits have changed.	4	2	1	0	0

Your Lifestyle

Circle the number for each statement that reflects your situation.

Column 1 = Always
Column 2 = Frequently
Column 3 = Occasionally
Column 4 = Rarely
Column 5 = Never

	1	2	3	4	5
You find time for daily, or almost daily, exercise.	0	0	2	3	5
You talk over your problems with your spouse, family members or friends.	0	0	2	5	7
You find time to read quietly, meditate, soak in the tub or listen to relaxing music.	0	0	2	5	7

Your Finances

Circle the number for each statement that reflects your feelings.

Column 1 = Always
Column 2 = Frequently
Column 3 = Occasionally
Column 4 = Rarely
Column 5 = Never

	1	2	3	4	5
You are concerned or angry you are making less money than you deserve to be making or your last raise was not enough.	18	16	8	1	0
You have financial problems because you don't earn enough money to support your family in the way you would like to.	15	13	5	2	0
You have a large mortgage that stretches your finances to meet each month.	8	6	4	2	0

Your Finances

Circle the number for each statement that reflects your situation.
Column 1 = 6 months ago
Column 2 = 1 year ago
Column 3 = 1-1/2 years ago
Column 4 = 2 years ago
Column 5 = 3 years ago

	COLUMNS				
	1	**2**	**3**	**4**	**5**
You declared bankruptcy.	10	8	6	3	0
Your mortgage or loans were foreclosed.	10	6	4	2	0
You took out large loans for cars, home improvements or other debts.	5	4	1	0	0
You paid college tuition.	4	3	2	0	0
You were sued.	8	6	5	2	0

INTERPRETING YOUR SCORE

To determine your score, add all scores from the categories. Check your total score below to see if your health and your life are at risk. You may be referred to the risk-reducing nutrition plan, page 186, or the risk-reducing exercise plan, page 226.

0 to 40   **Low Risk**—You are not under enough stress for it to be detrimental to your health.

41 to 60   **Moderate Risk**—You are under moderate stress but not enough to endanger your health unless you are subject to other risk factors that would compound your risk.

61 to 100   **High Risk**—You are under serious stress, which could damage your health. Take a look at your lifestyle and behavior patterns to see how you can take steps to help lower risks. The risk-reducing exercise plan and the risk-reducing nutrition plan will help lower your risk of stress-induced diseases.

100+   **Very High Risk**—You are under very high stress, and your health is in danger. Re-evaluate your goals and priorities, and adopt a less goal-oriented lifestyle. The risk-reducing exercise plan and the risk-reducing nutrition plan will help lower your risk of stress-induced diseases.

TAKE THIS TEST TO MEASURE YOUR
REACTION TO STRESS

This test measures whether your reaction to stress is detrimental to your health. Circle the score for each characteristic that applies to you. Total the score, then check your risk category on page 139.

Stress in Your Life

Circle the number for each statement that reflects your situation.

Column 1 = Always
Column 2 = Frequently
Column 3 = Occasionally
Column 4 = Rarely
Column 5 = Never

	COLUMNS				
	1	**2**	**3**	**4**	**5**
You point your finger or pound your fist for emphasis when talking.	5	4	3	1	0
You walk very fast and always seem in a hurry.	5	4	3	1	0
You talk so fast people ask you to slow down.	5	4	3	1	0
You do more than one thing at a time.	6	4	2	1	0
You interrupt other people or finish their sentences for them.	4	3	2	1	0
You jiggle your knee or tap you foot.	4	3	2	1	0
You make a point of being on time and are angry when others are late.	6	5	4	2	0
You eat fast and leave the table immediately after finishing your meal.	4	3	2	1	0
You must win and are competitive, even with children.	6	5	4	2	0
You get very impatient if kept waiting in line.	5	4	3	1	0
You get angry and impatient in stop-and-go traffic.	5	4	3	1	0
You lose your temper with other drivers.	5	4	3	1	0
You seethe with anger but don't show your feelings when someone crosses you, criticizes you or defeats you.	10	8	6	2	0
You lose your temper quickly when challenged, criticized or frustrated.	8	6	4	2	0

	COLUMNS				
	1	**2**	**3**	**4**	**5**
You become angry or irritable with your family when you are under pressure at work.	5	4	3	2	0
You make excuses for other people's inappropriate behavior or blame yourself for the incident.	5	4	3	2	0
You usually have more things to do than time to do them and worry you won't get everything done.	6	5	4	2	0
You say "yes" to more assignments or responsibilities even though you already have too much to do.	6	5	4	2	0
You ask for help when you need it.	0	0	1	2	3
You re-evaluate your activities or work and take steps to change your deadlines or priorities when you feel the pressure of having too much to do.	0	0	1	2	4
You are anxious about gaining approval for work you have done.	4	3	2	1	0
You are mainly interested in work and have no hobbies.	4	3	2	1	0
You often do things yourself because it's easier or you're the only one who can get it done right.	5	4	2	0	0
You relax with a drink to help get your mind off your problems.	4	3	2	1	0
If you smoke, you smoke more heavily when you're concentrating on a problem or when you're worried.	6	5	4	2	0
You use coffee or other caffeine-containing beverages or amphetamines to get you "up" for a difficult moment or day.	4	3	2	1	0
You use tranquilizers to help cope with stress, tension or symptoms of muscle spasms.	4	3	2	1	0
You take time each day, or almost every day, to sit quietly alone and purposefully relax your mind and muscles by a special technique, such as meditation, deep breathing, yoga or even listening to soft music.	0	0	3	4	5

	COLUMNS				
	1	**2**	**3**	**4**	**5**
You use a vigorous, competitive sport, such as racquetball or tennis, to work out your anger when you're upset.	7	5	3	1	0
You cope with personal problems by ignoring them and hoping they will go away.	7	5	3	1	0
You discuss your problems or worries with someone whom you can count on to listen and give you emotional support.	0	0	2	6	8
You try to please your friends or family, even though you feel unappreciated.	6	5	4	2	0
You give a lot more to friends or family than you receive.	6	5	4	2	0
You apologize when you make a mistake.	0	0	2	3	4
You blame yourself and worry when you make a mistake.	7	6	4	2	0
You comply with other people's wishes rather than your own.	7	6	4	2	0
You tell someone who has hurt your feelings you're hurt.	0	0	2	4	6
You smile and laugh often.	0	0	1	3	5
You make time for recreational activities or entertainment.	0	0	2	4	6

<u>INTERPRETING YOUR SCORE</u>

To determine your score, add all total scores. Check your total score below to see if your health and your life are at risk. You may be referred to the risk-reducing nutrition plan, page 186, and the risk-reducing exercise plan, page 226.

0 to 32   **Low Risk**—Your personality and the way you handle stress protects you from stress-related illnesses.

33 to 90   **Moderate Risk**—Your personality and the way you react to stress puts you at moderate risk of stress-related illnesses. Lower your risk by slowing your pace and learning better ways to cope with your problems.

91 to 147   **High Risk**—You are at high-risk of stress-related illness. Your personality traits and the way you cope with work-related and personal problems increase your risk needlessly. Learn to be easier on yourself; handle your problems by talking about them rather than ignoring them or losing your temper.

148+   **Very High Risk**—You are at very high risk of stress-related illness. Your personality traits and the way you cope with work-related and personal problems increase your risk. Expect a little less than perfection from yourself. Learn to share your problems by talking about them rather than ignoring them or losing your temper. Counter effects of stress with the risk-reducing exercise plan and the risk-reducing nutrition plan.

The Risk Factors of Stress

Emotional stress can affect your health as significantly as diet, smoking habits and exercise routine. Stress can be the risk factor that escalates the harm done by other outstanding risk factors that threaten your health. Your reaction to stress can damage your cardiovascular and cerebrovascular systems and lower your resistance to disease. Stress increases your chances of heart attack, stroke, sudden death and even cancer.

If you scored poorly on the stress risk-factor tests, think long and hard about your lifestyle and personality. It's possible to take positive steps to help eliminate the major stresses in your life or to make significant changes in the way you allow stress to affect you—changes that may be responsible for saving your health and your life.

Most of us define stress as a negative event or influence that is emotionally disturbing or disquieting. Positive events are also stressful—think of the heightened emotional state caused by a marriage, starting a new job, being selected for an award or being elected to an office. Whether positive or negative, stress affects your entire body because your emotions are communicated to your central nervous system, causing your adrenal glands to secrete hormones that prepare the body for action. The same hormones are secreted whether emotions are positive or negative, but more are secreted when you are negatively stressed.

Stress researchers frequently divide stress into three categories—cataclysmic events, personal events and background events. *Cataclysmic events* are unpredictable, powerful events that affect a large number of people, such as a war, earthquake or flood. *Personal events* happen to an individual or his family, such as death, accident, illness or job loss. *Background events* are daily hassles that are part of our everyday lives, such as traffic, noise, commuting, job dissatisfaction or family tensions.

You respond to all stresses in a similar way. Any stress triggers the same series of hormonal and behavioral responses. This response is called the *General Adaptation Syndrome,* a concept promoted by the well-respected stress researcher Hans Seyle. He believes you respond to any stress first with alarm, which sets off your hormonal response and activates the neuroendocrine system to a state of alertness. Then you begin to resist and cope with the stress until it is resolved. Repetition of stress, too many stresses occurring at once, stresses that cannot be resolved or poor coping mechanisms may lead to a state of exhaustion in which you can no longer cope with the stress. Once you reach the stage of exhaustion, the door may be opened to stress-induced diseases, such as anxiety, depression, high blood pressure, cardiovascular disease and cancer.

It is common for people to react to stress by becoming angry, hostile, depressed, even desperate. These reactions evoke a further response from your brain and central nervous system, causing them to release more stress hormones. The constant flow of these substances through the blood system, heart and brain is counterproductive to good mental and physical health. Over the years, continual stress may result in permanently elevated blood pressure, heart disease, stroke or cancer.

YOUR STRESS RESPONSE

During the alarm stage, your neuroendocrine system goes on the alert. The hypothalmus sends chemical messages from your brain to your adrenal glands, which respond with an outpouring of catecholamine hormones *epinephrine* (adrenalin) and *norepinephrine* (nor-adrenalin). These hormones step up your heart rate, raise your blood pressure, increase the conversion of stored energy to usable energy, reduce the blood flow to your skin and gastrointestinal tract but increase blood flow to your muscles.

When you are under stress, your adrenal glands are stimulated by the hypothalmus via the pituitary gland to secrete corticosteroid hormones, such as *cortisol,* which speed your body's access to stored fats and carbohydrates. Cortisol reduces tissue inflammation, causes an increased number of blood platelets, which are involved in blood clotting, and suppresses your immune system. Beta-endorphin, which diminishes pain, is also released.

This hormonal state of arousal was termed *flight or fight* by the pioneering stress researcher Walter Cannon in the early part of this century. It is a biological throwback as a reaction to danger. If you perceive a threat to your physical well-being, you must fight the attacker or flee from him. To do this successfully, your body gets geared up for action by sending more blood to your heart and muscles, increasing your blood pressure and preparing for a possible wound by increasing the blood-clotting factors. All these reactions serve a survival purpose if you are going to engage in a physical battle or run to safety at top speed. But if you are "threatened" by crowding on a subway, the constant noise of typing or worry over losing your job, you are neither fighting nor fleeing. The aroused state becomes a destructive force to your body and health.

Prepared for action, but going nowhere, your body reacts with heart palpitations, sweating, increased stomach acidity and spasm, and muscle spasms. Other chemical reactions take place in the body—the blood pressure rises, sometimes alarmingly, serum-cholesterol and fatty-acid levels rise, thrombosis-causing blood platelets increase, insulin secretion decreases and potassium and magnesium are wasted.

All of this activity can speed progression of hardening of the arteries everywhere in the body. Small, subtle, stress-induced foci of injury in the heart muscle can result in injury similar to that caused by an overt, painful heart attack. In addition to this kind of damage, norepinephrine secretion produced by anger and hostility can stimulate malignant rhythm disturbances in your heart in the form of ventricular fibrillation, the most common cause of sudden cardiac death.

Your body's reaction to a stressful event is useful only if you need to react physically to a threat—to fight or flee. Today's threats are usually of an emotional sort; the outpouring of hormones meant to prepare your body for physical battle is superfluous. Chronic stress damages your cardiovascular system, weakening your heart muscle, speeding up hardening of the arteries and causing rhythm disturbances in your heart's electrical system. Excessive corticosteroids may weaken your immune system, opening the door to cancer and other illnesses. Continual stress also leads to fatigue, anxiety and depression.

HOW STRESS AFFECTS YOUR HEART

Statistical analysis of many research studies clearly links high serum-cholesterol levels, high blood pressure, cigarette smoking and obesity to increased risk of heart disease. Yet many people without these risk factors have heart disease, as exhibited by angina pains, heart attacks and even sudden death. It has long been suspected that stress can harm the body's cardiovascular system, accounting for these cases of heart disease.

A dramatic reaction to stress occurs when someone "dies of grief." For example, this might happen to a man in good health a day after his wife's accidental death. His heart can't withstand the overload of stress hormones, primarily norepinephrine, that the blow of his wife's death dealt him. The excessive hormonal stimulation to the heart causes ventricular fibrillation, and he drops dead.

An example of the serious potential that "positive" stress can induce was revealed in a monitoring experiment on an otherwise healthy man who had a mild heart condition with occasional irregular heartbeats. He was hooked up to a heart monitor for an entire day. During the course of the working day, his irregularities were not alarming. That evening he attended an exciting New York Knicks' basketball game; as the game became more exciting, his heartbeats became more irregular. The game was won by 1 point in the last few moments; at the end of the game his heart rhythm exhibited a serious high-grade malignant rhythm disorder that did not subside until *4 hours* after the game was over. Fortunately, the rhythm disorder stopped short of the fatal ventricular fibrillation but only barely. His reaction was due strictly to emotional stress.

A dramatic reaction to another kind of stress was revealed in experiments done by Dr. Lawrence Hinkle of Cornell University. He monitored the heart rates and rhythms of people driving across town in New York City traffic. The results of the experiment showed an alarming incidence of serious heart-rhythm disturbances without the driver even being aware of the physical reaction that driving in such conditions was causing.

HOW STRESS AFFECTS CANCER

Several studies seem to indicate chronic stress can lead to cancer. Scientists believe the body's immune system constantly looks out for cancer cells and destroys them when they occur. Most of us probably produce cancerous or precancerous cells, but our immune system weeds out these cells and prevents them from reaching their deadly potential. If the immune system becomes weakened or damaged, these precancerous cells may grow out of control.

Stress can weaken the immune system. Studies of animals exposed to stress show damage to tissues of the immune system, such as the thymus, and an overall decrease in immune function. Crowded animals and animals exposed to stressful stimuli show an increase in cancer. Studies of identical twins, one of whom died of cancer while the other remained healthy, showed the twin with cancer had experienced more emotionally stressful life events.

Healthy students evaluated by Dr. Steven Locke at Beth Israel Hospital in Boston showed a marked decrease in function of the immune system if they reacted strongly to stress. Those who reacted to stress with a high level of psychological symptoms showed a significantly lower number of killer white blood cells circulating in their bloodstreams when compared to similarly stressed students who reacted less negatively to stress.

For 5 years, heavy smokers were followed by Dr. Margaret Linn at the Veteran's Administration in Miami to see who might develop lung cancer. Researchers recorded the same number of stressful life events—job loss, divorce, death in the family, major illness—among the lung-cancer victims as among those who remained healthy. The difference was that cancer victims found these events more stressful and blamed themselves more for their occurrences. Researchers found the immune-system response of the cancer patients was functioning poorly *before* the onset of cancer. This research shows that how you react to stress and how you cope with it are more important to your health and well-being than the amount of stress you experience.

TYPE-A, TYPE-B OR TYPE-C PERSONALITY?

Many researchers believe certain personality types are more susceptible to the harmful effects of stress. This reaction is probably due to coping style. Those of us who have learned to cope more successfully with stress rarely experience the state of exhaustion that can lead to fatal health effects.

The well-publicized *Type-A personality,* first described by San Francisco cardiologists Meyer Friedman and Ray Rosenman, is widely believed to be highly susceptible to heart disease. This person is characterized as being always under stress. He is highly impatient, easily angered, works long hours with intensity but never seems to have enough time to complete his work, self-critical and always on the run. Compulsively attracted to competition, the Type-A personality is usually very upset if he does not win.

Type-B personalities are relaxed, easygoing and laid back. The exact opposite of the Type-A person, the Type-B is thought to have a lowered risk of heart disease.

It is my experience that the Type-A person is not necessarily prone to heart disease and Type-B personalities are not necessarily protected from it. More subtle characteristics in some people—both Type-A and Type-B personalities—put them at risk.

Psychiatrists at Duke University recently concluded a key factor in the Type-A personality may be cynicism and hostility. Suspecting the Type-A behavior pattern might be too broadly defined, they set out to determine exactly what traits were linked most closely to fatal heart attacks. Those people who measured most cynical and hostile were 5 times more likely to have a fatal heart attack as those who had low scores for cynicism. People with these personality traits have been shown in laboratory experiments to produce more harmful hormones during a variety of experimentally stressful situations.

Behavior can be deceiving. Even if you are the kind of person who screams loudly at other drivers during rush hour or loses your temper when you have to wait in a long line, you may actually be unaffected inside—your adrenal glands do not necessarily react to a burst of temper by releasing stress hormones into your bloodstream. The outburst is more a learned behavior than a real reaction to stress. The external show of anger may be only external. It's really a matter of personality—some people use the show of emotion as a release and are actually much less disturbed than they seem. Other people perceive the stressful event as a personal attack, and stress hormones are released to do their destructive work on the body.

It follows that if you are a seemingly easygoing person who never shows his emotions on his face, you may actually be silently seething inside. If you are too controlled to show your anger or you repress your feelings, the anger simmers even longer, setting off reflexes from your mind through your neuroendocrine system to your glands, sending adrenalin and other hormones through the bloodstream.

A person who reacts to stress by silently seething—as opposed to the way a Type-A acts out his anger—is called a *hot reactor,* a term coined by Dr. Robert Eliot, a leading investigator of stress management. A hot-reactor may have either Type-A or Type-B personality behavior patterns and is probably more at risk than the Type-A whose reaction to stress is outwardly visible but inwardly not as dramatic. A hot-reactor with a Type-A personality is at the highest risk of heart disease.

Your outward reaction to stress can be deceiving, so it's important to learn to recognize the hidden symptoms of overreaction to stress. How can you tell whether you are a hot reactor? Tests can measure the body's physiological reactions to stress. For example, if a person who is a hot-reactor, with a normal blood pressure of 120/80, was hooked up to blood-pressure and pulse-measurement equipment and monitored while running on a treadmill, his blood pressure might rise to about 180/85 during the exercise and his pulse to 180. If he were also monitored while on the telephone in the course of an ordinary business day, his blood pressure might be found to go to 200/110 and his pulse to 120, merely from his reaction to the stress of doing business. The calm, efficient businessman may be revealed as a hot reactor—a person at risk of ill-health from his overreaction to stress.

It's unlikley your doctor can monitor you this way to evaluate your reaction to stress. But the stress-risk-factor tests can help you determine if you are at risk. If you are a hot-reactor, your personality traits may not give you away, but many symptoms caused by stress will.

People under stress often have gastrointestinal symptoms, such as constipation alternating with diarrhea, flatulence, indigestion or ulcers. They may have frequent headaches, muscle tension, especially in the back or neck, or they clench or grind their teeth. Behavior patterns that may not be recognizable to you are often recognizable to others. Be honest with yourself; listen to what other people have to say about you.

You can be evaluated at your doctor's office by the cold-pressor test, which was developed about 50 years ago but is just now gaining popularity. It is a very useful test that effectively distinguishes normal from abnormal vascular reactions to stress. Your hand is placed in ice water for 70 seconds, then your blood pressure is taken. If you are a hot reactor, your blood pressure will rise 20 to 50% above what it was just prior to the ice-water treatment. If you are not a hot reactor, your blood pressure will rise no more than 10%.

Another method of evaluating reaction to stress involves playing mental games, such as repeatedly subtracting 7s beginning with the number 777 in a limited time period. A skilled evaluator can tell from observing the way you react to this mental game or how you play a competitive video game or answer a series of questions what your temperament is and what your internal reactions are to the stresses. These games set up reactions similar to the responses to fear, anxiety, anger and hostility.

You can test yourself by taking your pulse immediately after an emotionally stressful event, such as a disagreement with your spouse, a long wait in the supermarket line or driving in heavy traffic. Then take your pulse again 1/2 hour later. Whether you are a Type-A who acts out your anger or a hot-reactor who simmers inside, your pulse will be racing about 30% faster than usual even 1/2 hour later because of your overreaction to the stressful event. Observe whether or not your palms are perspiring, you are pale, whether or not your stomach feels tied in knots or if you have a dull headache—these are also signs of stress.

Some researchers speculate that there may be a *Type-C personality*—this personality type is more susceptible to cancer. As I discussed earlier, a lowered immune response as a result of stress can lead to cancer. According to research by Dr. Lawrence LeShan published in the *Journal of the National Cancer Institute*, cancer victims seem to have some prominent personality traits in common. These people:

- Give more than they receive in personal relationships.
- Comply with wishes and demands of others rather than their own needs.
- Set up emotional barriers to forming close relationships.
- Feel they are unworthy of love.
- Have a "Pollyanna" outlook on life.
- Repress real anxieties and appear to be strong, well-adjusted and coping well while actually they are emotionally insecure.
- Feel an unusual amount of self-pity.
- Had an unhappy, stressful childhood.
- Are loners without an extensive social-support system.
- Sweat the small things.

The Type-C personality puts on a happy face while he lives with insecurity, loneliness and self-pity. The stress induced by trying to be someone you're not, by repressing true feelings and failing to form a close supportive network of friends and family takes its toll on the immune system. An oversupply of corticosteroid hormones is produced, which may make you more susceptible to cancer.

HOW TO IDENTIFY STRESS

As researchers study stress, some surprising insights about stress and how to deal with it have been revealed. By comparing researchers' findings with your own life situation, you can identify the harmful stresses in your life and take positive steps to eliminate them.

The competitive workplace and the business world are seen by many of us as breeding grounds for stress-induced diseases. This may be true for some of us, but others seem to thrive on the stress. What explains this?

Let's take a look at two seemingly stressful lives. Which of the following two people—SLB or FJM—would you consider to be under more stress, and why?

SLB is the 50-year-old newly appointed president of a large corporation who was brought on board to solve looming financial and mismanagement problems. He has had to relocate his family, buy a new house and is sending his oldest child to college, with the other two not far behind. He travels a lot and puts in long hours. His wife is bored and lonely in the new city.

FJM is a 50-year-old junior executive of a large corporation where he has worked for 20 years. There has been a massive reorganization of the company that has left him with reduced responsibilities, so there is little pressure to perform on the job. Because of this, he has plenty of time to spend with his wife and two teenage sons. His wife has a good job and the mortgage is practically paid off, so he has no immediate financial worries.

On the surface, it would seem that SLB is under more stress on the job and at home.

But FJM is probably under greater stress because he feels bored, useless and angry at work and at home. His career seems to have dead-ended. He has no power at work and worries he may be fired in the next reorganization. He feels like a failure, and he is angry that after all his dedication to the company he is getting squeezed out. He worries he may lose his job entirely and no other company would hire him, so he wastes time trying to look busy and needed. His wife's career seems more exciting than his, and she is too busy to spend much time with him. He is concerned he has lost face with her and his sons because of his seeming demotion. Though there are no present financial problems, FJM worries if he is fired his wife will have to support the family, and he hasn't saved enough money for his children's college tuition.

Though SLB's job is very demanding and everyone expects him to perform miracles, it's a great ego booster. He feels confident and powerful. People listen to him and do what he says. He is seeing positive results from his long hours of work and feels good about himself. He is paid a huge salary and knows even if he doesn't succeed in turning the company around there will be another good job and salary elsewhere. His relationship with his wife needs some attention, but he has money enough to take the family on vacation to the Caribbean at Christmas and to lavishly furnish their new home.

The important point these examples make is that harmful effects of stress are often due more to your reaction to stress than to the stress itself. If you feel you have control over your life and the stresses involved, you will fare better. If the end result of a stressful situation is to build your self-esteem, you are less stressed. Hard work and long hours are not as stressful if you feel positive about your job. If your long hours are productive and you are praised for your hard work, this adds to your self-esteem.

But if the long hours are frustrating and your hard work unappreciated, the stress level increases greatly. Doing nothing all day and feeling discouraged about being able to improve your situation (as was the case with FJM) is extremely stressful.

Experiments with animals and human subjects demonstrate the importance of control over stress and reaction to the stress. Animals that are able to control when stress, such as an electrical shock, occurs show less stress-induced conditions than animals subjected to the same amount of electrical shock delivered randomly. Human subjects who are told they can control the volume of a loud noise or the degree of an electrical shock, when they actually have no control, are less stressed than those who are told they have no control.

As women's roles have changed in society, there has been concern that they are opening themselves up to the stress-induced diseases that affect men. In fact, the rate of heart disease among women has risen during the past several decades. I attribute this to the increase in cigarette smoking and the use of birth-control pills and estrogen replacement rather than to stressful jobs.

Researchers from Columbia University, Princeton University and the Wellesley Center for Research on Women have shown the home may be the most stressful place for women. Women who are at home all day with young children are more depressed and anxious than their husbands who work. A woman who has an interesting job, a husband and children is usually happier than her jobless counterpart. Women playing up to five roles, such as wife, mother, part-time worker, volunteer and student, exhibit better mental health than those with fewer roles—unless the women's roles are wife, mother and provider. These women report considerable stress, perhaps because they are carrying the full financial burden and working at an unrewarding job.

This research supports the theory that demanding jobs are not as stressful as they might seem if they build self-esteem. The job of being a mother to two toddlers is only rewarding in the long-run. On a day-to-day basis, it doesn't build self-esteem and is often isolating, repetitive and boring. The mother who can get out of the house and get involved in an interesting job or activity that builds her self-esteem is doing herself good rather than adding more stress to her life by taking on more responsibilities.

Women who are forced to work at menial jobs for financial reasons and who would rather be at home with their children are under considerable stress. It is again a matter of control. The woman who is doing what she wants to do, rather than what her husband or society thinks she should be doing, is under the least emotional stress.

Cataclysmic events can cause stress, but an earthquake, hurricane or war may be less stressful in the long-run than other events. Researchers believe that even though the aftereffects of cataclysmic events are felt for years, several factors make them less stressful than we might expect.

A severe earthquake involves large numbers of people and is catastrophic in its damage, but the actual threat from the earthquake is brief, then social forces seem to take over. People work together to rebuild, and they give each other moral support. We cope with disaster, even severe loss of life and property, by believing the worst is over and better days are ahead. Hope and hard work give us the illusion of control.

A personal disaster, such as a spouse's death or loss of a job, can be as strong and unexpected as an earthquake, but it affects fewer people. Unless you have a close, supportive network of family and friends, you won't have anyone to share your disaster with. Without this coping mechanism, a personal loss could be more stressful to you than a destructive earthquake in which you lose your home.

If you have friends and family to give you proper emotional support and have learned effective coping mechanisms, you will begin to recover from your personal disaster, though it may leave scars for years. Things will gradually improve and because the severest point of the stress was brief and behind you, there is hope for recovery. You reassess your skills and goals and go out and aggressively look for a new job. You gain new interests, become active in the community or suddenly fall in love again. With encouragement of friends and family, you draw on your own resources and give yourself hope for a better future and a feeling of control.

Daily hassles or worries, called *background stressors,* may not seem like much at first. Constant low-level noise or numerous unexpected loud noises, commuting, crowding, family tensions and job worries may be persistent problems that don't seem overwhelmingly important. They are not dramatic or life-threatening, but they never seem to go away; you feel as if you have no control over them. When many low-intensity stresses are added together, they can have a very high-intensity effect.

Constant noise takes its toll. Studies show noise can trigger the flight-or-fight response. Your heart beats faster, your blood pressure rises and your digestive system slows down. This kind of background stress makes you more irritable, tired and depressed. Add the stress of the noise of your workplace to the stress of working with a person you don't like or to the stress of not sleeping well because you have a new baby, and you increase your stress level considerably.

The combination of enough background stressors may leave you unable to cope, and you reach your stress-exhaustion level without understanding why. Chronic background stresses are difficult to cope with because you feel as if you have no control over them. You can't assure yourself the worst is over and things are getting better—you may even feel they're getting worse. You can't rely on the emotional support of your family and friends the way you can when you experience a personal crisis. Your coping mechanisms become easily exhausted. You lose your ability to cope with even the most trivial stresses, losing your temper easily at home and at work. Combine background stresses with a major personal stress, and you increase your risk of heart disease, cancer and other illnesses.

YOU CAN REDUCE STRESS

We know overreaction to stress, rather than the nature of the stress itself, damages health. To lower your risk from stress you must learn some different behavior patterns and coping mechanisms. If you learn good coping skills, the major and minor stresses of life won't break you down.

If you have an overreactive Type-A personality, you *can* and *should* change your behavior. Recent research by Dr. Meyer Friedman shows among heart-attack victims with Type-A behavior, those who were taught to modify their personalities had a significant reduction in second heart attacks. All the heart-attack victims were given standard advice about diet and exercise, but only some of them participated in group therapy designed to modify Type-A behavior. Three years later, those in the behavior-modification group had only half the risk of heart attack as the other group.

To modify your Type-A behavior, make an effort not to turn petty annoyances of life into major crises. Every time you feel yourself hassled, mad or time pressured, stop and ask yourself if your reaction is worthy of the event. Does it really matter if you are 10 minutes late for your appointment? So what if you got caught at a red light? What difference does it make if you get beaten at racquetball? Take a few deep breaths, and make a conscious effort to relax.

Type-A people must also learn to stop driving themselves so hard. You must look at

149

your life and decide what is really important as a life goal. Concentrate on what you'd like to be rather than on what you'd like to have. Understand and admit you can't accomplish everything. Decide what's most important, then try to work toward that goal rather than 10 goals at once.

Ask yourself how much of what you're doing is simply to conform to the pressures of society, your co-workers, your friends and your family. Keep in mind that your lifetime is limited; decide what you *really* wish to accomplish and which activities are really important to you if your life were to end sooner than you expect. If you don't like what you're doing, make changes so you're doing what you like.

Reduce your hostility and competitiveness toward others because these traits seem to be some of the key risk factors of Type-A behavior. Learn to be more accepting of other people and your own shortcomings. The Type-A should make a consistent effort to try the following:

- Be friendly, and smile at strangers.
- Do good deeds.
- Give another driver the right of way.
- Let someone else win a competitive game on purpose.
- Let someone go in front in line.
- Overlook a minor mistake by a co-worker instead of rubbing it in.

As you learn to accept others for who they are, you'll accept yourself more. If you can't make these changes on your own, seek professional help. Group therapy designed to modify Type-A behavior seems more successful than individual psychological counseling.

Support systems are important. Whether you are a Type-A or a Type-C personality or a hot reactor, you may need to put more energy into your personal relationships and friendships. If you are a hard-driving overachiever, it's likely you direct energy into your career that should be put toward your personal life. Research has shown those who have family and friends to help them through a crisis fare much better than those who don't. Consider how much you give and how much you take from other people. You'll be happier and more fulfilled if you can rely on other people in times of personal crisis.

If you are naturally reticent and insecure and bottle your feelings inside, it's a good idea to seek professional counseling to help you overcome these traits. Only by learning to reach out and express your true feelings to others can you overcome your Type-C or hot-reactor personality. Therapy can help you develop the self-esteem and self-confidence you need to help you get more from your relationships.

Don't take your family and spouse for granted. Giving them your love also means giving them your time and energy. But having a good marriage should not mean giving up your own individuality because that may lead to frustration, anger and hostility.

When you feel yourself reacting to physical or emotional stress, make an effort to dissipate the stress. This may mean taking a few deep breaths and relaxing your tense neck, back or jaw muscles. You may also try meditating for 10 minutes by sitting still with your eyes closed, breathing deeply and trying to think of a relaxing image. Even rocking in a rocking chair has proven beneficial for some people. Biofeedback has its place in stress therapy if you need help learning to relax.

Drugs sometimes play a role in stress control if you are at high risk of heart attack. But tranquilizers are overused in this country to smooth out problems instead of curing them. This type of medication is useful in the short term, but in the long term it creates greater stress by solving nothing. To be constructive, drug use must be professionally supervised.

Beta-blockers block the heart from reacting to norepinephrine. They can play a major role in protecting people with known heart conditions from the effects of stress. Your doctor can advise you which beta-blocker is right for you, if such a drug is necessary.

Don't depend on alcohol to cope with stress. You can't hide unhappiness with alcohol—it complicates and worsens the problem. Heavy alcohol consumption is a risk factor of heart disease, stroke and cancer. Why compound your risk by coupling overreaction to stress with alcohol use?

Exercise is an excellent way to reduce stress. It helps burn up excess stress hormones in your bloodstream and helps relax tense muscles. Some researchers even claim exercise causes the release of mood-elevating endorphin hormones, which might explain why people who exercise regularly feel good.

Don't use hard exercise as an outlet for angry or hostile emotions because you may do yourself more harm. Taking a long, brisk walk can help release the tensions of a stressful work day, but don't begin a vigorous activity, such as rowing or racquetball, while you are seething with anger. Exercise adds to the excess demands being made on your overstimulated system.

Don't exercise immediately after smoking, and never exercise under the influence of stimulating drugs, such as amphetamines, excess coffee or alcohol. These chemical influences produce excess norepinephrine, which can overstimulate the heart. The normal heart *almost always* withstands extra stimulation, but a heart that is compromised with the beginning of atherosclerosis might experience a malignant arrhythmia.

One of my patients had a hot temper, and one evening he had a fierce argument with his wife. She walked out on him. He drank alcohol to soothe his anger, then ate a big meal. Because he was so distraught, he took sleeping pills to calm himself down and slept through the night. He awakened with renewed anger and went out for his daily jog. Half-way through his run, he dropped dead of cardiac arrest due to malignant arrhythmia. His stress-induced cardiovascular reaction would probably not have happened if he hadn't added to his stress with drugs, alcohol and vigorous exercise.

If the personal and background stresses of your life are building up to overload level, you can lower your risk by taking positive steps toward change. Concentrate on your family and friends rather than on material things in your life. Become more accepting and tolerant. Slow down and enjoy life; don't be in such a hurry to get where you're going. What you're hurrying toward might just turn out to be a premature death from cancer, heart disease or stroke!

For maximum risk reduction, combine lifestyle and personality changes with the risk-reducing exercise plan, page 226, and the risk-reducing nutrition plan, page 186. By exercising, you can dissipate the stress hormones that may be damaging your cardiovascular and immune systems. A diet rich in grains, fruits and vegetables, and low in fat and cholesterol builds a healthy heart and immune system, capable of fighting off cardiovascular disease and cancer. Stress reduction, combined with a nutritious diet and exercise plan, helps reduce your risks.

12.
THE RISKS FACTORS OF POOR NUTRITION

TAKE THIS TEST TO MEASURE YOUR
NUTRITION KNOWLEDGE

This test measures your level of knowledge about nutrition. There is one correct answer for each question. Check your answers against the correct answers beginning on page 157, then check your score on page 161.

NUTRITION QUESTIONS

1. Assuming you eat three balanced meals a day, which would make the best snack?
   a. Cheese and crackers
   b. Peanut butter and crackers
   c. 1 medium banana
   d. 8 ounces of orange juice
2. Which of the foods listed below has the most protein per ounce?
   a. Flounder
   b. Ground sirloin
   c. Cheddar cheese
   d. Low-fat (1%) milk

3. Which food has more calories ounce for ounce?
    a. Baked potato
    b. Rib-eye steak
    c. Vanilla ice cream
    d. Creamed cottage cheese
4. There's more nutritional value in which of the following foods?
    a. Apple juice
    b. Fresh apple
    c. Applesauce
    d. They're equally nutritious
5. Which food has more fiber per serving?
    a. Cucumber
    b. Lettuce
    c. Banana
    d. Apple
6. Which vegetable is the most nutritional source of calcium?
    a. Celery
    b. Potato
    c. Broccoli
    d. Spinach
7. Which "dietetic" lunch is most nutritious and also low in calories?
    a. A 3-ounce hamburger patty, 1/2 cup low-fat cottage cheese and 1/2 cup fruit salad.
    b. 1 slice whole-wheat bread and salad of 1/4 avocado, 3-1/2 ounces iceberg lettuce, 3 ounces water-packed albacore tuna and 1/4 large green pepper.
    c. 2 slices whole-wheat bread with 1 teaspoon margarine, 1/2 cup low-fat cottage cheese with 1/2 cup cantalope and 1 medium-sized fresh peach.
    d. 2 slices whole-wheat toast and 6 ounces strawberry-flavored low-fat yogurt.
8. The most well-balanced, nutritious breakfast is:
    a. 2 poached eggs, 2 strips crisp bacon, 2 slices whole-wheat toast with 2 teaspoons of margarine and 4 ounces orange juice.
    b. 2/3 cup 40% Bran Flakes, with 1 cup sliced fresh strawberries and 8 ounces low-fat (1%) milk, and 2 slices whole-wheat toast with 2 teaspoons margarine.
    c. 3 pancakes with 3 tablespoons maple syrup, 2 sausage links and 4 ounces orange juice.
    d. 2 poached eggs, 4 ounces hash-brown potatoes (fried in vegetable oil), 2 slices whole-wheat toast with 2 teaspoons margarine and 6 ounces orange juice.

9. Which of the following foods is the most nutritious source of vitamin C?
   a. Banana
   b. Green pepper
   c. Spinach
   d. Acorn squash
10. Which of the following vegetables is *not* in the cabbage family?
    a. Cauliflower
    b. Broccoli
    c. Kale
    d. Spinach
11. Which of the following statements about pasta is *true?*
    a. Pasta is a high complex-carbohydrate food and should be eaten in limited quantities because it's fattening.
    b. It's all right to eat pasta if you buy the protein-enriched brands.
    c. Pasta is a nutritious, high-complex-carbohydrate food and may be eaten frequently if it isn't prepared with cream-based sauces.
    d. Pasta should be eaten with cream-based sauces to complement the protein.
12. Which one of the following vegetable oils is saturated?
    a. Cottonseed oil
    b. Safflower oil
    c. Coconut oil
    d. Sesame oil
13. Which statement about vitamins is true?
    a. Don't worry about taking too many vitamins because your body excretes whatever it doesn't need.
    b. If you eat enriched bread, you don't need vitamin pills.
    c. If you eat a balanced diet, you don't need vitamin pills.
    d. Even if you eat a balanced diet you should take vitamin pills as a kind of insurance policy.
14. Which statement about fast food is true?
    a. Chicken nuggets or fish filets contain more fat than a regular hamburger.
    b. French fries are usually cooked in lard.
    c. A vanilla shake contains more sodium than a regular serving of French fries.
    d. All of the above.
15. Which of the following statements is true?
    a. If eaten in the right combinations, vegetables and grains can provide a good source of protein.
    b. The only good sources of protein are meat, fish and dairy products.
    c. Eggs are a nutritious, low-fat source of protein.
    d. None of the above.

16. Which of the following foods contains the most calcium?
    a. 1 cup of skim milk
    b. 1 cup of whole milk
    c. 1 cup of cottage cheese
    d. They all contain the same amount of calcium
17. Which of the following foods is the most nutritious source of vitamin A?
    a. Broccoli
    b. Carrots
    c. Spinach
    d. Acorn squash
18. Which of the following statements is true?
    a. Enriched white bread is more nutritious than whole-wheat bread.
    b. Enriched white bread is as nutritious as whole-wheat bread.
    c. Whole-wheat bread is more nutritious than enriched white bread.
    d. Whole-wheat bread contains more bran but fewer vitamins than enriched white bread.
19. One egg yolk contains:
    a. 275mg cholesterol
    b. 125mg cholesterol
    c. 320mg cholesterol
    d. 0mg cholesterol; cholesterol is in the egg white.
20. How many medium-sized shrimp contain the same amount of cholesterol as one egg?
    a. 5
    b. 10
    c. 15
    d. 20
21. How many grams of fiber should you eat every day to help reduce risks of various diseases?
    a. 8
    b. 15
    c. 30
    d. 40
22. A 12-ounce can of Pepsi Cola contains how much sugar?
    a. 5 teaspoons
    b. 8 teaspoons
    c. 10 teaspoons
    d. 12 teaspoons
23. Polyunsaturated fats should be:
    a. Eaten freely because they are good for your heart.
    b. Severely restricted in your diet because they may cause stomach cancer.

    c. Eaten moderately because too much fat can cause cancer.

    d. Eaten freely because they prevent heart disease and cancer.

24. Which fish contain protective omega-3 fatty acids?

    a. Salmon

    b. Tuna

    c. Scallops

    d. All of the above

25. The amount of alchohol contained in two 5-ounce glasses of wine is equal to how much 80-proof liquor?

    a. 1 shot (1.5 ounces)

    b. 2 shots (3 ounces)

    c. 3 shots (4.5 ounces)

    d. 4 shots (6 ounces)

ANSWERS TO NUTRITION QUIZ

1. The correct answer is c. A banana is the best choice because it provides complex carbohydrates, vitamins and fiber without unnecessary fat. A medium-sized banana contains 105 calories, which are mostly complex carbohydrates.

   Although an 8-ounce glass of reconstituted orange juice (answer d) contains vitamins and about the same number of calories as the banana (112 calories), the calories come mostly from sugar. Sugars are readily absorbed into your bloodstream and quickly raise your blood sugar level but don't satisfy your hunger for long.

   Cheese and crackers (answer a) and peanut butter and crackers (answer b) are high-fat, high-calorie snacks. One ounce of cheddar and three Ritz crackers contain 168 calories—65% from fat. One ounce of creamy peanut butter and three Ritz crackers contain 149 calories—67% from fat.

2. The correct answer is a. Flounder has the most protein per calorie. A poached flounder filet is 87% protein; the remainder of the calories come from fat. A broiled ground sirloin hamburger (answer b) is 49% protein; the remaining calories come from fat.

   Cheddar cheese (answer c) is 56% protein. The remaining calories come primarily from fat.

   Low-fat (1%) milk (answer d) is 70% protein; the remaining calories come primarily from carbohydrates.

3. The correct answer is b. The rib-eye steak has more calories; each ounce contains about 71 calories.

   Each ounce of baked potato (answer a) contains about 25 calories.

Each ounce of vanilla ice cream (answer c) contains about 57 calories.

Each ounce of creamed cottage cheese (answer d) contains about 30 calories.

4. The correct answer is b. The fresh apple contains the most fiber and takes longest to digest, which causes a less-rapid increase in blood sugar levels than do the juice or sauce. Calorie for calorie, the fresh apple provides almost 2-1/2 times the amount of fiber as the applesauce and juice.

5. The correct answer is d. An apple has the most fiber. A medium-sized apple with the skin has 1.1 grams of fiber.

   A medium banana (answer c) has 0.6 grams of fiber.

   Half a medium cucumber (answer a) with the skin has 0.3 grams (without the skin 0.2 grams).

   A 3-1/2-ounce serving of lettuce (answer b) has 0.5 grams of fiber.

6. The correct answer is a. One large stalk (3-1/2 ounces) of cooked broccoli contains 88mg of calcium.

   Two stalks (3-1/2 ounces) of raw celery (answer a) contain 40mg of calcium.

   One medium-sized baked potato (answer b) contains 9mg of calcium.

   1/2 cup of cooked spinach (answer d) contains 83mg of calcium, but most of this is bound in a chemical form unavailable to your body.

7. The correct answer is c. All the lunches contain about 350 calories, but the most nutritious is Lunch C because it is the most nutritionally balanced. It contains 384 calories—20% from fat, 58% from carbohydrates and 22% from protein—a nutritious mix in a weight-loss diet.

   Lunch A, a hamburger pattie, cottage cheese and fruit salad, is low in fiber and too high in saturated fat and protein, which may increase cancer and heart disease risks. It contains 368 calories—39% from fat, 21% from carbohydrates and 40% from protein.

   Lunch B is also high in fat (unsaturated from the avocado) and protein but provides plenty of fiber and vitamins from the fresh vegetables. The lunch contains 350 calories—45% from fat, 23% from carbohydrates and 32% from protein.

   Lunch D is a high-carbohydrate meal that contains 343 calories—12.5% from fat, 74.7% from carbohydrates and 15.8% from protein. But it is not as nutritious as Lunch C because it provides no vitamins from fruit or vegetables (the strawberry flavoring doesn't count), and it is too low in fat to meet the body's needs.

8. The correct answer is b. Breakfast B is the most nutritious because it contains 27% fat, 57% carbohydrate and 17% protein, and no cholesterol. There's plenty of fiber and vitamins from the whole grains and fruit.

   Breakfast A has 470 calories but is high in fat and cholesterol. It contains 52% fat, 31% carbohydrates and 17% protein, with almost twice the recommended daily allowance of cholesterol.

Breakfast C has 946 calories and is too high in calories and fat. It contains 43% fat (saturated fat from the sausage), 41% carbohydrates and 16% protein. The cholesterol is twice the recommended *daily* amount.

Breakfast D has 629 calories—46% fat, 41% carbohydrates and 13% protein. It contains almost twice the recommended *daily* amount of cholesterol.

9. The correct answer is b. Green pepper is the best source of vitamin C—64mg in half a large green pepper.

    A medium-sized banana (answer a) contains 10mg of vitamin C.

    1/2 cup of cooked spinach (answer c) contains 25mg of vitamin C.

    1/2 cup of baked acorn squash (answer d) contains 13mg of vitamin C.

10. The correct answer is d. Spinach is not in the cabbage family. The other three vegetables belong to the cabbage family and contain a substance that researchers believe may be protective against colon cancer.

11. The correct answer is c. Pasta is nutritious and provides protein and carbohydrates without fat. It is not high in calories unless eaten in excess or eaten in dishes with cream or cheese-based sauces. For full protein complementarity, combine pasta with beans, a small amount of meat or low-fat dairy products.

12. The correct answer is c. Coconut oil is saturated. The other vegetable oils are unsaturated.

13. The correct answer is c. Vitamins are unnecessary if you eat a balanced diet and have no unusual health problems. Vitamins in excess can be harmful to your health.

14. The correct answer is d. All of the statements about fast foods are true. Chicken and fish are fried and contain more fat than a regular hamburger. The breading on chicken often contains ground chicken skins, adding additional saturated fat and cholesterol.

    Lard (a saturated animal fat) is often used for frying fast food.

    A vanilla shake contains 201mg of sodium, and French fries contain 101mg of sodium.

15. The correct answer is a. If combined properly so all essential amino acids are included in the same meal, vegetables and grains do not provide unneeded fat. Meat, fish and dairy products (answer b) are good sources of protein, but they often contain too much fat.

    The protein in egg white (answer a) is considered an almost-perfect protein (with an excellent balance of amino acids), but the egg yolk contains close to the daily limit of cholesterol, making it an unnutritious protein source on a regular basis for most people.

16. The correct answer is a. Skim milk contains 302mg of calcium per cup. Whole milk (answer b) contains 288mg of calcium per cup.

    Cottage cheese (answer c) contains 138mg of calcium per cup.

17. The correct answer is d. All these foods are good sources of vitamin A, but acorn squash is the best. One cup of acorn squash contains 172% of the minimum daily requirement of vitamin A.

    A cup of cooked broccoli (answer a) contains 95% of the minimum daily requirement of vitamin A.

    One cup of cooked carrots (answer b) contains 159% of the minimum daily requirement of vitamin A.

    One cup of raw spinach (answer 6) contains 89% of the minimum daily requirement of vitamin A.

18. The correct answer is c. Whole-wheat bread is the most nutritious because it contains fiber, vitamins, protein and carbohydrates.

    White bread contains only a trace of fiber, whether it is enriched or not, and does not contain all the vitamins found in whole-wheat bread.

19. The correct answer is a. One large egg yolk contains 275mg of cholesterol.

20. The correct answer is d. One medium-sized shrimp contains about 14mg of cholesterol; 20 medium-sized shrimp equal the 275mg of cholesterol in one large egg.

21. The correct answer is c. Thirty grams of fiber a day, which is more than we consume on the average, seems to provide protection against colon cancer.

22. The correct answer is c. There are 10 teaspoons of sugar in a can of Pepsi Cola.

23. The correct answer is c. A balance between saturated, polyunsaturated and monounsaturated fats gives the best protection from cancer.

24. The correct answer is d. All these fish contain fats that may be protective against heart disease.

25. The correct answer is b. Two shots (3 ounces) of liquor contain the same amount of alcohol as 10 ounces of wine.

INTERPRETING YOUR SCORE

To determine your score, add up the number of *wrong* answers. Check your total score below to determine your level of understanding about nutrition.

11 +   **Poor Knowledge**—Your knowledge of nutrition is based more on myth than fact. Because of this, you may not be eating as nutritiously as you could, and you may be putting your health at risk.

6 to 10   **Moderate Knowledge**—Your knowledge of nutrition is better than average, but you still subscribe to some fallacies. If you improve your understanding of the food you eat, you may reduce your health risks.

3 to 5   **Good Knowledge**—Your knowledge of nutrition is good, but there is still room for improvement. Decide where there are gaps in your understanding and learn the facts.

2 to 0   **Excellent Knowledge**—Your knowledge of nutrition is excellent. You answered nearly all the questions correctly; as long as you practice what you know, you are protecting your health.

The Risk Factors of Poor Nutrition

Evidence is steadily mounting that what we eat plays a major role in our long-term health. Heart disease, cancer, high blood pressure and diabetes may be avoidable—*if* we eat properly. If we overeat and don't follow a nutritious, well-balanced diet, we may be encouraging these and other serious illnesses to shorten our lives.

We have one of the world's most abundant, varied food supplies, yet we often eat foods that are bad for our health. We should be the best-fed population in the world, but we are often overfed and undernourished at the same time. We eat "junk food" that supplies our bodies mainly with empty calories, fat, sodium and caffeine, without supplying us with the nutrients we need for good health.

If you choose foods laden with calories from refined sugars and fats, but which lack vitamins and minerals, you may gain weight without being properly nourished. You may suffer from deficiency diseases even though you're overweight.

Eating has lost its primary purpose—to nourish the body—and has become almost a purely self-indulgent, pleasurable pursuit. This is fine if the foods that taste good are also the foods that are good for you. But our palates have been trained to respond so strongly to salt and sugar that peaches canned in heavy syrup taste better to many than the real thing ripened on a tree! Many people prefer cola over a glass of milk. We eat corn chips, candy bars and pretzels as snacks instead of nuts and fruits. We eat hot dogs and hamburgers rather than fresh seafood and chicken breasts. We eat white bread instead of whole-grain bread and sugared cereals instead of oatmeal.

Your goal should be good nutrition, but satisfying your palate needn't be an afterthought if you educate yourself to appreciate the good taste of nutritious foods.

If you nourish your body, you'll be supplying the fuel and building materials needed so your body functions best for the longest possible time. The better nourished you are, the better your body will serve you—mentally and physically. The better you'll feel, and the longer you'll feel that way. By eating a nutritious diet, you'll avoid harming your body with excesses or imbalances. You'll avoid foods that are harmful and eat foods that protect your body from disease.

Your body is a complex machine; it won't stop immediately if you fail to give it the best kind of fuel and maintenance, but over time, and perhaps without warning, it will stop—the works will be gummed up and the parts worn out. Care for your body properly, and it will run efficiently for a long time.

In designing an ideal diet to protect you from disease and keep you trim and fit for a lifetime, you must strive for the following:

- Achieve a nutritious balance between proteins, fats and carbohydrates.
- Eat a variety of foods.
- Avoid foods that are harmful.
- Emphasize foods that are protective.
- Create a diet that appeals to your palate.

My sound, nutritious, risk-reducing nutrition plan, page 186, combines *all* these desirable features at once. It provides you with needed calories and nutrients while it reduces the risk factors of heart disease and cancer. It helps control weight and satisfies your taste buds. Satisfaction and taste must not be given first priority if satisfaction means sugar, fat and salt, which it often does for many of us. I believe one of the main reasons millions suffer from heart disease, high blood pressure, cancer and obesity is because we have eaten a non-nutritious but "tasty" diet.

It's possible to lower your health risks if you eat more nutritiously. If you change your ways gradually, it won't be difficult to make the necessary adjustments in your diet to achieve good nutrition and enjoy your food at the same time.

You are probably familiar with protein, carbohydrates and fats, but I am amazed at the misconceptions people have about them. Often my patients are unsure about what foods provide which nutrients, and misconceptions abound. A little review seems in order.

FATS

Every day, your body needs fat in the diet. Dietary fats provide energy needed to perform normal physical activity because fat is burned along with carbohydrates for energy. Dietary fat helps you absorb important vitamins, such as the fat-soluble vitamins A, D and E. The layering of your body with appropriate amounts of fat is one of Nature's ways of protecting internal organs from injury. This layering also helps maintain body heat.

You can fulfill all your body's fat requirements on a low-fat diet, but you must understand which fats to eat. Some kinds of fats are better for you than other kinds, so you must learn which they are and how much is safe to eat.

Dietary fat can be *saturated* or *unsaturated*. Animal fats are usually saturated, and vegetable fats are usually unsaturated. Saturated fats are solid at room temperature, and unsaturated fats are liquid at room temperature. Unsaturated fats may be very unsaturated, called *polyunsaturated*, or slightly unsaturated, called *monounsaturated*. Oils that are *hydrogenated*, a process that makes them more solid at room temperature, have hydrogen added to the fat molecule, making it more solid and more saturated. This is done in making margarine and vegetable shortening.

Saturated fat in excess is statistically associated with increased risks of heart disease and certain cancers, such as cancers of the colon, breast, pancreas and prostate. Saturated fats are found in whole-milk dairy products, such as cream, butter, cheese and whole milk, and in the fat in poultry skin and red meat.

Polyunsaturated and monounsaturated fats in the diet are associated with a lower risk of heart disease. These fats come primarily from vegetable oil, nuts, seeds and margarine. Whole-grain breads and cereals, and vegetables contain a small amount of unsaturated fat. The oils and fats in plants are usually unsaturated, except for palm oil and coconut oil—they are saturated, and you should avoid them. Olive oil and avocado have high amounts of monounsaturated fat.

Cholesterol is a sterol with many properties of a fat, and it is carried in a compound called a *lipoprotein.* Cholesterol is found in large amounts in egg yolks, meat fat and whole-milk dairy products. Saturated fat is found in most of the foods that contain high levels of cholesterol.

Your body needs cholesterol to make hormones and cell membranes, but your liver makes all the cholesterol you require. Excess cholesterol in the diet is associated with vascular and heart disease. The higher your serum-cholesterol level, the greater your risk of cardiovascular disease, so a diet low in cholesterol is advisable.

Saturated fats in the diet raise serum-cholesterol levels; unsaturated fats lower them. Until recently, polyunsaturated fats were considered the most effective cholesterol fighters. Recently, new evidence indicates that monounsaturated fats are also effective cholesterol fighters. Monounsaturated fats, such as olive oil, were shown by researchers at the University of Texas to lower overall cholesterol levels by lowering heart-damaging LDL cholesterol in relation to protective HDL cholesterol.

PROTEINS

Proteins are complex nitrogen-containing molecules built from subunits called *amino acids.* There are 22 amino acids that can be strung together in a limitless arrangement; the arrangement determines the particular protein. Your body needs all 22 amino acids and can convert some amino acids into other kinds. But it can't manufacture eight amino acids; these *must* be included in your diet. These eight amino acids are called *essential amino acids.*

Every cell in your body contains protein, and you need a small daily supply of protein to maintain bodily functions and cellular repair. Fortunately, many foods contain protein, and it is utilized slowly. The breakdown of protein into individual amino acids is a complicated chemical process and happens more slowly than the carbohydrate breakdown. The amount of protein we need on a daily basis is small, and this amount may decrease as we get older.

Your body can't store protein or amino acids as protein, and that's the reason you need some protein every day. Your body converts any excess protein into fat or glycogen (a complex storage sugar) that your body burns for energy. Excess nitrogen left after this conversion is excreted in the urine.

Animal protein contains the essential amino acids in almost the same proportions that your body needs; this type of protein is called a *complete protein.* Soybean protein is also a complete protein. Its pattern of amino acids conforms closely to that of milk.

Most plant foods are *incomplete proteins,* which means they are short on one or two of the three limiting amino acids—tryptophan, lysine and methionine. All eight amino acids are equally essential, but the three limiting amino acids are most often found in inadequate amounts. If you get enough of these in the foods you eat, you'll get the necessary amounts of all the other essential amino acids. The three limiting amino acids are the keys to protein completeness.

Some plant foods have large amounts of the amino acids in which other plant foods are deficient. The foods complement each other's deficiencies and are used to supplement one another. Combined in the right proportions, they make up a source of high-quality protein. When used together, foods like corn and beans, whole-wheat bread and milk, beans and rice, peanut butter and whole-wheat bread, or tortillas and beans are high-quality, complete-protein sources. Their combined amino-acid pattern has no deficiencies. Another example is rice and wheat, which are limited in lysine but contain sufficient amounts of methionine. When rice or wheat is combined with beans or legumes, which are low in methionine and have sufficient lysine, you have a complete protein.

On the risk-reducing nutrition plan, you reduce the amount of animal protein in your diet and increase the amount of plant protein. To help you nutritionally, you will need to become aware of how to make a complete protein. You may have to spend some time and make an effort to learn how to combine protein sources for completeness, but any effort you make now will be worth it in the long run.

Relying on vegetables as the *primary* source of protein is healthier than relying on meat as the primary source. Meat protein is almost always accompanied by fat, and fat is the dietary culprit responsible for increasing your risk for numerous diseases. Some meats actually have 4 times as much fat as protein! Including a small amount of meat in your diet helps balance the vegetable protein.

CARBOHYDRATES

Carbohydrates are made of carbon, hydrogen and oxygen, and they fall into two basic groups: *simple carbohydrates* and *complex carbohydrates*. Simple carbohydrates are sugars made of one molecule (monosaccharide) or two molecules (disaccharide). Complex carbohydrates are starches made of chains of monosaccharides (polysaccharides) and are the primary storage foods of plants. Fibers, which give plants structure and strength, are also polysaccharides.

Your digestive system transforms most carbohydrates into their component simple sugars, which are absorbed by the bloodstream and converted by the liver into the blood sugar *glucose*. Once you've digested a carbohydrate food, it's utilized immediately for energy or converted to glycogen and stored in your liver and muscles to be used as a quick energy source and a blood-sugar regulator. Your body converts excess glucose into body fat.

Natural sugars and starches, eaten in unprocessed or minimally processed foods, such as fresh fruits, baked potatoes, steamed rice, beans and frozen or fresh vegetables, are good for you. These starchy foods should be the mainstay of your diet; they provide complex carbohydrates and small amounts of protein. When combined correctly with each other or with small portions of dairy or meat protein, vegetable protein becomes balanced.

Your body can't digest some polysaccharides in fruits, vegetables and grains, but they aren't wasted. These polysaccharides, such as *cellulose, pectin, hemicellulose* and *lignin,* are collectively called *fiber.* Fiber passes through your digestive tract undigested, adding bulk to bowel movements. Fiber helps keep the fats and cholesterol you eat from being totally absorbed and helps speed any carcinogens in your system through your digestive system.

Absence of adequate amounts of fiber can cause constipation, diverticulitis and appendicitis, and it can increase your risk of colon and breast cancer. Eating adequate amounts of fiber offers some protection from these diseases and may also lower serum-cholesterol levels because fiber prevents dietary fat from being digested and absorbed. Oat-bran fiber appears to enhance excretion of cholesterol, other sterols and bile acids, so it may offer some protection from cardiovascular disease.

VITAMINS

The word *vitamin* sounds like "vitality" and suggests an importance in providing energy. But vitamins provide no energy. Their importance lies in their role as co-factors in the many chemical reactions that take place in your body.

Vitamins are essential to the chains of chemical reactions that manufacture genetic material, blood cells and hormones. Your body needs a very small amount of each vitamin; if you eat a balanced diet, you probably won't lack any essential vitamins.

Many people take supplementary doses hoping to ensure continued good health. Vitamins from a balanced diet are in correct proportion and are better absorbed by the body when they come from food rather than from pills. Vitamin supplements are generally unnecessary. Your body excretes the excess in your urine or stores extra amounts in body fat, which can lead to toxicity.

Many food faddists advocate the use of megadoses of vitamins. There is evidence certain vitamins may be protective against cancer, but evidence does *not* indicate that megadoses are needed. Megadoses can be very dangerous and cause imbalances in other vitamins and minerals in your body. Don't take them!

The incidence of true vitamin deficiency in our society is low, except in people on extreme or unusual diets. Vitamin supplements are warranted only in special cases, such as illness, a bad smoking habit, excessive use of alcohol, use of birth-control pills or unconventional diets. Excessive intake of polyunsaturated fats may create the need for a little more vitamin E in smokers or those who live in smoggy areas. These people may benefit from 30 units of vitamin E a day, but over 400 units is likely to cause fatigue. A woman who takes birth-control pills may be deficient in folic acid and should take supplements of folic acid upon the advice of her physician.

Marginal vitamin deficiencies do occur in people who do not eat balanced diets, especially if a diet lacks fruits and vegetables. But these deficiencies can usually be corrected by dietary adjustments. That's the safest solution. If you increase your intake of fresh fruits and vegetables, you'll probably feel much better.

If you feel the need to take vitamins because you've been eating poorly or if you're a heavy smoker or drinker, you might safely take a multivitamin supplement for a month or so. Take only the recommended daily dose, not megadoses! Read labels, and select a balanced multivitamin produced by a recognized pharmaceutical company. Drug companies have spent millions of dollars in research to come up with a pill that balances vitamins in the right proportion to each other and in the right dosage. Never take large doses of a single vitamin!

I cannot emphasize enough that a well-balanced diet should supply all the vitamins your body needs. If you feel you'd benefit from taking a certain vitamin, for whatever reason, talk with your doctor. Large doses of vitamins can be toxic and should be taken *only* under the supervision of a physician.

Vitamin overdoses can cause many problems. Recently one of my patients (a prominent actor), came to me complaining of swollen feet and a miserable, itchy red rash all over his body. After much questioning, I discovered his wife was trying to nurse him back to health after a bad illness by giving him large doses of B-complex vitamins. These had caused kidney, blood-vessel and skin problems, which accounted for his symptoms. I told him to stop the excess vitamins immediately, and after a few weeks the symptoms were gone.

We take $3 billion worth of unnecessary vitamins a year. In many cases, people take more than 20 times the amount their bodies need. This can create serious imbalances and can damage the body's ability to store or absorb vitamins. Increases in one group of vitamins is not the key to reducing risk of disease because this "solution" causes other problems.

Excess vitamin C may result in a washout of vitamin B-12, creating a deficiency. Taking 1,000 to 2,000mg of vitamin C a day, which is 10 to 20 times the amount your body requires, creates the need for additional vitamin B-12 and iron. Both are washed out of your body in the urine, along with the excess vitamin C, which your body rejects as unnecessary.

When you stop taking large doses of vitamin C that your body has become accustomed to, you may find you have developed a permanent need for megadoses. You must wean yourself off this high level. I believe taking more than 1,000mg of vitamin C is excessive. It is doubtful vitamin C will help you avoid or cure a cold—no matter how well-publicized this "fact" is. Research does not support it. Excessive vitamin C may create kidney stones; in pregnant women it may cause scurvy in newborn babies.

Megadoses of vitamin A (over 25,000 units a day) can result in liver toxicity, skin discoloration, headaches, blurred vison, overgrowth of certain bones, drowsiness, headaches, nausea and vomiting. These effects are reversible, but frequently the diagnosis is delayed because the user assumes only positive results are possible from taking a vitamin supplement.

Health faddists often promote the vitamin-B-complex group, which includes thiamin, riboflavin, niacin and B-6 (pyridoxin), as a way to renew vitality in people under stress. Your body requires only 20mg of niacin and about 2mg a day of these other vitamins. Some popular vitamin mixtures contain 10 to 20 times this amount. When taken in high doses, problems with the liver, brain, skin, kidney and blood vessels may develop.

The major benefit of vitamin E and its publicity in recent years has been to manufacturers, not its users. Excess vitamin E can actually cause thrombophlebitis (clotting in the vein), a condition it is meant to cure.

If competent researchers prove the benefits of certain vitamins or minerals as an aid to longevity, the news won't be kept secret. You'll hear about it on radio and TV and read about it in the newspapers. But unconfirmed theories belong in laboratories with experimental animals—not in your bloodstream or jumbling your brain cells.

MINERALS

Inorganic substances—iron, calcium, potassium, manganese, chromium, flouride, zinc, magnesium, phosphorous, sodium, copper, selenium—also play an important role in your health. Your body needs these substances only in small quantities. With the exception of iron, phosphorous and calcium, it is unlikely anyone who eats a balanced diet will be deficient in these substances.

Growing children and women who are pregnant or who menstruate heavily may be iron-deficient. Nutritionists have recently revised their thinking about the need for calcium in older women. It's unlikely anyone following a basic nutritious diet needs extra mineral supplementation.

The same warnings for excessive use of vitamins apply to minerals. A varied, balanced diet supplies all the essential minerals your body needs. Megadosing with minerals, such as zinc and selenium, can be very dangerous, causing your system to become unbalanced and depleting it of other essential minerals or even poisoning your body. Your body has only a certain capacity to adapt to excesses.

Zinc has gained unfounded popularity as a mineral to improve sexual performance. This myth began when research showed zinc fed to infertile rats—ones that had been bred to be infertile—showed increased fertility. Fertility and sexual competence are not the same, but the media and pseudo-nutritionists responded by labeling zinc as a sex potion. Sales of zinc soared. In large amounts, zinc causes an imbalance in copper utilization by the body—an imbalance that hastens the progression of arteriosclerosis.

Many of us consume sodium in great excess. Your body needs only 200mg of sodium a day, although the National Academy of Sciences recommends 1,100mg daily. The average American gets 5,000 to 7,000mg of sodium every day from his food. A healthy person can safely eat 2,000 to 2,500mg a day, but in susceptible people, even this amount may raise blood pressure. A quarter teaspoon of salt contains about 500mg of sodium; each serving of processed food you eat contains much more than that—read labels!

Sodium is present naturally in our food, but it is also found in table salt, sodium bicarbonate, baking soda and some brands of antacids. Canned food (sodium is used to maintain the taste in canning and processing), processed meat, cheese, MSG, pickles and processed foods are also high in sodium.

Excess dietary sodium is a major cause of high blood pressure. Your body maintains a balance of sodium, potassium, calcium and magnesium. This biochemical equilibrium is hampered when the ratio of sodium is too high, resulting in water retention. In certain cases, excess sodium causes loss of magnesium and potassium from the cells, which may cause serious heart-rhythm disturbances. The sodium-potassium ratio is vital to good muscle function, kidney efficiency and heart function. The key is to avoid excessive amounts of sodium. A balanced diet without added salt will take care of your sodium needs, and your system will work optimally.

Our typical diet relies too much on high-calorie foods and doesn't include enough fresh fruits and vegetables. It lacks fiber and contains too much fat and animal protein.

It's possible to eat well and enjoy your food while preventing diet-caused diseases. My risk-reducing nutrition plan can help reduce the incidence of heart attack and cancer. Try it—you may live longer and feel younger!

13.
THE RISKS OF FAD DIETS

Every day in the United States, more than 50 million people are trying to lose weight on some type of diet. But the frustrating fact is that most people won't be able to keep off the weight they lose. More than 95% of all dieters who try quick-weight-loss diets regain the weight they lose. More alarming, quick-weight-loss diets are hazardous to your health. They are usually nutritionally unsound and may promote heart disease, kidney disease, cancer and even sudden death. Lesser side effects include fatigue, irritability, constipation and diarrhea.

If you quickly regain weight you lost on a fad diet, you'll probably try to shed the pounds again. This causes yo-yoing up and down in weight, which may be more of a health risk than carrying around a few extra pounds.

Fad diets are hard to resist; they promise to solve all your weight problems in short order. The diet tells you what to eat and when the diet is over. For example, the Scarsdale Diet or the Beverly Hills Diet rely on specific quantities or types of food that you eat for a specific number of weeks. In return for your adherence to the miracle combination of foods, each promises a quick weight loss.

These diets often guarantee a weight loss of as much as 10 to 14 pounds in a couple of weeks. But the weight almost never stays off, even if you manage to follow the diet faithfully and shed the pounds. The reason these diets fail when it comes to permanent weight loss is they are designed to cause rapid weight loss by radically, sometimes dangerously, tampering with your metabolism. The initial weight loss is water loss not body fat.

Many people who desperately want to lose weight follow a fad diet for longer than they are advised to and put themselves at even greater risk. You may do great harm to your health following these diets even for the suggested time limit.

Quick-weight-loss diets have one thing in common. They promise you won't feel hungry or deprived because you can eat as much as you want of certain food items—meat, in the case of some, and fruit, in the case of others. In reality, they are all low-calorie diets. This fact is hidden from you, and you are told weight loss is due to some chemical or physiological change in your body induced by this miraculous combination of foods. The appeal of the diet is you believe you'll lose weight fast—usually within 2 or 3 weeks—and you won't feel hungry because the diet lets you eat tasty things.

This appeals to many people. If you like to eat and are overweight, you probably have little tolerance to the prolonged frustration that accompanies cutting off the pleasures of eating. You fall for the premise of the diet, no matter how scientifically unsound it may be. You convince yourself that after the diet you'll be able to maintain your weight loss, but you resume your old eating habits.

THE HEALTH RISKS OF FAD DIETS

Many fad diets are high-protein, low-carbohydrate diets. They appeal to the common misconception that carbohydrates are fattening. They don't admit it, but many of these diets are also high in fat because fat comes hidden in meat protein. These diets go against all basic health principles of balanced, nutritious eating. High-protein, low-carbohydrate diets may increase your risk of cardiovascular disease and cancer. Your cholesterol level may rise dramatically because of excessive amounts of animal fat; this increases your risk of heart disease. The lack of carbohydrates and fiber, along with excessive fat, increases your risk of colon and breast cancers.

The case history of one of my patients, JMS, is a good example of the harm that can be done on one of these diets. JMS was a 49-year-old male, 5' 10'' tall, who weighed 196 pounds. He tried to lose weight by following a high-protein, high-fat, low-carbohydrate diet with vitamin supplements. The chart below shows his weight loss over an 8-week period and the dangerous changes in his body's blood chemistry that accompanied the weight loss.

Week	Weight	Cholesterol	HDL	Triglycerides
Start	196lb	197mg/dl	52mg/dl	89mg/dl
4	178lb	222mg/dl	48mg/dl	195mg/dl
8	168lb	265mg/dl	39mg/dl	222mg/dl
% Change	− 14%	+ 25%	− 25%	+ 125%

It looks as though the diet was successful. In 8 weeks, JMS lost 28 pounds, an average of 4-1/2 pounds a week. But blood tests reveal a different scenario. His cholesterol, HDL and triglyceride levels changed from acceptable levels to risky levels, which increased his risk of cardiovascular disease.

After dieting for 8 weeks and losing 28 pounds, JMS was irritable, constipated and unable to sleep or concentrate. He stopped the diet and 10 weeks later weighed 192 pounds. His risk factors of heart disease were elevated beyond what they had been before he started the diet because of elevated cholesterol and triglycerides. This case is a common occurrence for many people embarking on crash diets.

I convinced JMS to try a long-term diet, similar to the permanent weight-loss diet I describe on page 204. He followed the plan for 16 weeks, eating a balanced diet of 1,200 to 1,400 calories a day without any vitamin supplements. The chart below shows the happy results of the program.

Week	Weight	Cholesterol	HDL	Triglycerides
Start	192lb	222mg/dl	45mg/dl	155mg/dl
4	188lb	222mg/dl	47mg/dl	115mg/dl
8	185lb	212mg/dl	52mg/dl	122mg/dl
12	181lb	197mg/dl	51mg/dl	98mg/dl
16	177lb	201mg/dl	54mg/dl	95mg/dl
% Change	-8%	-20%	+18%	-30%

JMS lost 15 pounds, and he felt good—better than he had in years. More importantly, along with the weight loss, his blood cholesterol and triglyceride levels dropped significantly, and his protective HDL level rose. JMS has kept his weight under control for 4 years.

The side effects JMS suffered are not the only health hazards of quick-weight-loss diets—risks can be considerably greater. They range from dizziness, nausea, hypotension (low blood pressure), diarrhea, fatigue and irritability (all of which you might willingly tolerate to lose those annoying pounds), to cardiac disrhythmias, kidney failure and stroke. These complications should convince you to try another method of weight loss.

You lose weight initially on a high-protein, low-carbohydrate diet because the nutritional imbalance causes your body to get energy from fat calories not carbohydrate calories. This results in an accumulation of toxic-breakdown products called *ketone bodies* in your blood. This state, called *ketosis,* leads to nausea, vomiting, fatigue, dizziness and low blood pressure.

Ketosis is dangerous to your health. It interferes with your metabolic pathways, respiratory system and kidneys, and your blood's acid-alkaline balance is upset. The ketosis cycle causes cells to lose water first into the bloodstream, then through the kidneys. Ketosis creates an unhealthy state that induces dehydration and electrolyte depletion.

Your body metabolizes at a specific rate to support lean body tissue. When tissue is lost, your metabolic rate slows down, making further weight loss more difficult. The long-term results of this overall slowdown can be traumatic and serious. Personality changes, such as depression, and other changes, such as slowed reflexes, irritability, insomnia, poor concentration and bowel disturbances, may result because of ketosis-induced altered metabolism.

A high-protein diet stresses your kidneys by causing them to excrete excess nitrogen from digested protein along with fluid. This is noticed as a dramatic weight loss. (Over 60% of the weight you lose on such diets is water.) Low-carbohydrate diets also raise your blood's uric-acid level, which may lead to gout or kidney stones. The diets may also cause constipation.

10 FAD DIETS

There are many popular fad diets that have appealing or flashy names. Every year at least one or two diet books make the best-seller list. Many of these diets can be harmful to your health and do not result in permanent weight loss. The list on pages 174 and 175 details some of the more-popular diets that have been promoted in recent years. Though marketed as radically different from each other, these diets each reduce caloric intake but not in a balanced, nutritionally safe way.

If you read and analyze any of these diet books, you can see how fallacious the diets are. The Beverly Hills Diet, which was promoted a few years ago, is nutritionally absurd. The book is rampant with unscientific statements, such as undigested food "gets stuck in the stomach, thus causing weight gain." The book states many concepts that contradict established biochemical facts.

The Beverly Hills diet is based on eating nothing but fresh fruit. Fruit is nutritious, but without any major sources of fat and protein, the diet is dangerously unbalanced. The distorted consumption of fruit can cause severe diarrhea, leading to fluid loss, sodium and potassium deficiency, low-fluid-volume shock, cardiac arrhythmias and muscle weakness. You lose weight by diarrhea and breakdown of lean body tissue.

The Scarsdale Diet and Cambridge Diet are low-calorie, ketogenic diets, deficient in minerals, vitamin A and riboflavin. They cause quick weight loss by inducing ketosis because of the low-carbohydrate, high-protein, high-fat content.

Many people tried liquid-protein diets several years ago, and drank nothing but the prescribed number of ounces of diet food. More than 40 people died before the FDA took the liquid protein off the market.

The fad diets listed on the following pages aren't the only unhealthy diets people have been gullible enough to follow. From macrobiotics to starvation, from Stillman to F-Plan, people have tried these because they wanted a rapid, permanent weight loss without long-term diet control. As long as you subscribe to this propaganda, you'll *never* permanently lose weight.

THE BEVERLY HILLS DIET

Premise: The right combination of fresh fruits provides enzymes that unlock ugly fat from your body—eat nothing but fruit for 6 weeks, including expensive tropical fruit.

Enzyme theory is scientifically unfounded. Any weight lost initially is water from diarrhea and urination caused by excessive fruit. *Muscle,* not fat, is broken down to provide energy in this diet, which is deficient in calcium, iron, niacin, protein and fat.

THE IMMUNE-POWER DIET

Premise: On the Scarsdale Medical Diet, Dr. Atkins' Diet and Calories Don't Count Diet, you can eat generous portions of meat and/or vegetables and still lose weight without counting calories.

Allergy theory is unfounded. You will lose weight on this diet because it is a *low-calorie* diet. It is fairly well-balanced but deficient in calcium.

THE HIGH-PROTEIN AND HIGH-FAT DIETS

Premise: In the Scarsdale Medical Diet, Dr. Atkins' Diet and Calories Don't Count Diet, you can eat generous portions of meat and/or vegetables and still lose weight without counting calories.

These are low-calorie, high-protein, high-fat diets. Scarsdale provides about 1,100 calories a day, much of it from large portions of meat. You lose weight rapidly and temporarily because of fluid loss and the dangerous state of ketosis. There is possible kidney, respiratory and nervous-system damage from ketosis. Heart damage may result from excess fat.

THE PRITIKIN DIET

Premise: This high-carbohydrate, very low-fat, low-protein diet will reverse degenerative diseases and help you shed pounds.

The diet is 5 to 10% fat, 10 to 15% protein and 80% complex carbohydrates, which is very difficult to follow. It is too low in fat, resulting in deficiency of essential fatty acids and fat-soluble vitamins A, D, E and K. Adherence may result in protein deficiency because no proper guidelines are given on combining plant proteins. Calcium, zinc, iron and copper deficiencies are due to excess chemicals in plant foods that combine with these minerals, making them insolute. The diet is so extreme that most people are incapable of following it for any prolonged period, leaving the dieter feeling guilty when he cheats.

THE CAMBRIDGE DIET & THE LAST-CHANCE DIET

Premise: This special concoction of liquid protein results in weight-loss without calorie counting.

These are near-starvation diets with dangerous side effects, such as heart arrhythmias, serious dehydration, fatigue, hair loss and bowel dysfunction. They have caused at least 40 deaths from ketosis. Both diets are vitamin deficient, and the Last-Chance diet is protein deficient.

THE F-PLAN DIET

Premise: Increasing fiber in your diet will fill you up and keep you from overeating. You'll lose weight without counting calories.

Excessive fiber can cause flatulence and deficiencies in calcium, zinc, copper and iron. Weight is lost because this is a low-calorie diet in disguise.

THE FIT FOR LIFE DIET

Premise: We are fat because the food we eat "clogs" our systems and is inefficiently eliminated. To unclog the system and lose weight, you must eat food that is 70% water because your body is made of 70% water. Overweight results from breaking the natural laws of life and eating the wrong combinations of foods. Eating nothing but fresh fruit all morning cleanses your system of toxic wastes and frees up energy to help you lose weight.

You lose weight on this diet because it's a low-calorie diet. Explanations of digestion and nutrition are fallacious. The diet may result in vitamin, protein, iron and calcium deficiencies—the authors even admit your hair and fingernails may fall out.

WHY FAD DIETS FAIL TO KEEP WEIGHT OFF

If your desire to lose weight by some quick-loss scheme is undaunted by the potential health risks these diets pose, consider the following. As soon as you stop the diet, the ketotic condition ends, and the water weight comes back. Within a few days you may gain back as much as 60% of what you lost! Dehydrated cells are like a dried sponge; they suck up water from any food or fluid you ingest. The weight you lost is quickly regained. The on-again, off-again patterns of quick-weight-loss diets encourage food binges and rapid weight gain. For long-term weight control, these diets are self-defeating.

Quick-weight-loss diets are not nutritionally balanced because they concentrate heavily on foods you might not normally eat. After you finish dieting, you don't know what to do next. A fad diet leaves you without long-term guidance—it's designed only for the short-term. You often return to your former eating habits and weight-gaining foods.

Once you gain the weight back, you probably blame yourself. You believe in the diet, so the failure must be yours. You and your family and friends may believe it's your fault and you have no willpower. You lost the weight, but you didn't have the willpower to stop overeating—that's why you gained it all back. This isn't true! It's not your lack of willpower; it's the fraudulent premise of the quick-weight-loss diet that did you in.

Crash diets don't help you change eating patterns that made you overweight in the first place. Your eating pattern isn't unbreakable, but you need guidance to change it, or you'll never lose weight permanently.

Some psychoanalysts assume overeating is "just a habit" or a gratification of oral needs, but it's more than that. Overeating is a means of using food to relate to the world, to enjoy the world or defend yourself from it. If you use food as a weapon against anxiety or depression, as many overweight people do, dieting increases the stress in your life. By depriving yourself of food, you thrust yourself into distressing situations without any "protection."

In this battle, diets are merely token acts. You may attempt to lose weight to please someone else, but you never achieve the goal. Only when you learn coping mechanisms other than opening the refrigerator to eat whatever is in there will you be able to face the world without a food pacifier. Only when dependency on food as a symbol of security ends will you be able to lose weight and keep it off.

Most people don't recognize or contend with this aspect of dieting. Instead they repeatedly attempt an assortment of quick-weight-loss fad diets with sad results. The overweight person hates to be called "obese." He minimizes the relationship between the amount of food he eats and the weight he gains. If you're overweight and addicted to a pattern of eating that is hard to break, choosing the quick solution offered by fad diets will never work for you. You can't hand over the responsibility for your condition to anyone offering a new gimmick.

The gimmick won't work, and you'll shop around for the next miracle diet. You must admit to yourself these diets are good only for the short term as a convenient rationalization for your failure to permanently change your eating habits. These diets are a convenient way of avoiding the real reasons for your overweight.

SHOULD YOU DIET?

For many people who are 15 to 20% over their ideal body weight, quick-weight-loss diets will probably fail. A mild excess in overweight is not recommended, but it is better than harming your health with fad diets. If you're more than 20% overweight, your health is already at risk—that's all the more reason not to go on an unbalanced diet that carries increased risks of a variety of diseases, including cardiovascular disease, diabetes, carbohydrate intolerance, reduced life span and sudden death.

If your choice is to diet, it must be to diet *successfully!* If your reason for dieting is to fit into a new summer wardrobe, chances are your diet will only be successful for the summer. If you want to diet successfully and permanently, you must reach a point where being overweight is no longer acceptable to you. You have to face up to the need to change a pattern of eating, not for 2 weeks or 2 months, but permanently. To make this permanent adjustment, you have to carefully examine your goals and understand what they are. Before you can diet successfully, you need to understand *why* you have failed in the past to lose weight and keep it off. You first must understand why you are overweight.

Understanding the habits that made you overweight and changing them provides the clue to keeping the weight off forever. Crash diets fail to help you deal with the reasons behind your excess pounds. The causes of overweight are not well-defined; in some cases, psychosocial problems and a poor self-image conspire to create an overeater who continues to suffer in a cycle of unsuccessful yo-yo weight-loss diets. Other evidence suggests overweight is of genetic origin in some cases.

A glance at the history of overeaters and chronic dieters reveals interesting patterns. Some people become addicted to food after a long record of overeating because they believe "eating well is healthy." That slogan, in one form or another, has been imposed on many of us.

Do you remember what your mother said when you didn't finish everything on your plate? Can you recall what you felt? Remember what it was like when you finished everything on your plate—you pleased your mother, and that made you feel good. The association of food with a desire to please became firmly ingrained. Obedience relieved the anxiety produced by the rejection that accompanied not finishing your meal. When you told your mother, "I'm not hungry," you created pressure. That tension was alleviated by eating, whether or not you were hungry.

Over the years, you began to realize the pleasant sensation related to eating could neutralize anxiety—at least temporarily. Food, particularly sweets, can become a perfect "drug" against anxiety and depression. Overeaters become addicted to food, and they use it as a way to cope with stress or anxiety.

Being overweight makes exercise less pleasant than for normal-weight people—it encourages a less-active lifestyle. This lower level of activity causes further weight gain and may make weight loss even more difficult.

Shedding extra pounds is difficult. By losing weight—and giving up the pleasure of eating—you may gain social acceptance. But the price is high and uses a lot of emotional energy. Frequently the short-term gratification of eating overwhelms the long-range goal of looking better and gaining social acceptance. One is immediate and real; the other too distant and too indefinite.

I believe one reason many of us are overweight is because we are hooked on empty-calorie "junk" foods. This food lacks nutrients and is loaded with sugar, fat and sodium. As children, we often develop a taste for these foods that stays with us throughout our lives. Many of us feel a meal isn't complete without dessert. Beverages don't taste good unless they're sweet. When we're hungry, we want to eat satisfying foods rather than what is good for us. Parents often bribed us with sweets, which became a reward and an emotionally loaded food. We were encouraged to eat our meat (loaded with fat calories) if we wanted dessert.

Another situation is overweight that creeps up on us as we grow older. For many people, the battle for weight stability during the teen years is lost in the years from 20 to 40. Dr. Theodore Van Itallie of Columbia University and Dr. Albert Stunkard of the University of Pennsylvania, well-known researchers in the field of obesity, believe obesity that develops during early adulthood (between 20 and 40) may be a greater health hazard than overweight carried from childhood.

The body may adjust to lifelong overweight, but excessive weight gained in midlife may result from sudden, unhealthy changes in eating habits or from stress. The body may not be able to adapt to the additional excess weight.

With the years, our bodies automatically slow down; we need fewer calories to maintain our weight. Of those over age 30, more than 40% of the men and 50% of the women are at least 10% over suggested weights. This propensity toward weight gain as we age combines with the tendency to develop other unhealthy conditions to increase our overall risk of ill-health. But the physical risks that overweight may cause are not the only reasons for concern. The lethargy and low self-esteem many obese or overweight people feel may be the result of obesity, not its cause.

Research indicates some people may be born to be fat. The size and number of fat cells varies from person to person, but the number of fat cells doesn't usually change much during your life—only the *size* of the cells changes. People who are heavy beginning in childhood have a larger number of adipose (fat) cells in their bodies. Even after losing weight, they easily gain because those fat cells are waiting to blow up again.

A clinical investigation of actual fat tissue in women with lower-body obesity shows their fat cells are normal size, but there is an excessive number of cells because of overeating during growth and childhood. In upper-body fat, the pattern is reversed; cells are normal in number but larger because of overeating during adulthood.

The larger-than-normal size of fat cells caused by excessive weight gains in adulthood increases the risk of adult-onset diabetes because fat cells have insulin receptors on their surfaces. There are fewer receptors in the same volume of fat made up of large cells compared to fat made of normal-sized cells. This reduction in the number of insulin receptors causes the body to produce more insulin to compensate for the lower number of receptors. In people genetically predisposed to diabetes, overeating during adult life can lead to adult-onset diabetes.

Dr. Jules Hirsch from Rockefeller University believes the number of fat cells is determined around age 2. It is important for infants and young children to maintain a healthy weight. Chubby babies may be cute, but they may also have lifelong weight problems. A toddler regularly given an extra helping of ice cream to pacify him or a preschooler introduced to soft drinks and candy bars may develop habits and tastes that will be difficult to reverse as he grows older. Examine the regularity with which you or your children were exposed to this sort of treatment. You will be amazed at how widespread these seemingly innocent practices are.

Studies of identical twins further support the idea weight may be genetic, at least in part. When raised separately, identical twins' body weight as teenagers and adults tends to be relatively consistent. The frequency of obesity in certain families further supports the theory that a tendency to overweight may be genetic. Some researchers believe overweight people may be born with defective neurotransmitters in their brains. These defects may result in an inability to recognize the point of satiation. They will overeat without realizing their appetite has been satisfied.

The causes of overweight are complex. In many people, psychosocial problems and a poor self-image conspire to create an overeater who continues to suffer through life in a cycle of unsuccessful dieting. Many obese people became overweight because they ate too many non-nutritious calories—candy, cake, soft drinks or alcohol—that provided empty calories.

Because you burn calories during your tennis workout or other exercise, you tell yourself you're getting energy from junk food, so it's all right to eat it. This is a rationalization because the amount of exercise is probably insufficient to burn off the number of calories consumed. The result is weight gain.

When you eat, consider the nutritional benefits other than calories that you derive from your food choices. Most people, especially those who are overweight, greatly underestimate the number of calories they consume.

You *can* lose weight safely and keep it off. The trick fad diets play on your body—the unnatural release of body fluid and water—is only a temporary weight loss. Few people who follow these diets sustain any degree of successful weight loss. Even though you may be serious about losing weight, by choosing a fad diet you only prolong your overweight.

If you are sincere about losing weight, but have always been unsuccessful, the permanent weight-loss diet should work for you—if you're committed. It provides you with sound nutrition, healthy exercise and intelligent calorie counting. I can't promise you'll lose 10 pounds in a week, but you will be gratified to see the pounds shed slowly and steadily, and you should be able to keep the excess weight off permanently.

PART II.

RISK-REDUCING PROGRAMS

14.

FEEL YOUNGER, LIVE LONGER

A long, fulfilling, healthy life can be yours if you take steps now to lower your health risks. The risk-reducing nutrition plan, page 186, and the risk-reducing exercise plan, page 226, will put you on the road to good health. If you need to lose weight, you can do so successfully, permanently and safely with the weight-loss diet plan. See page 204. If stress is increasing your health risks and decreasing the enjoyment you should be getting out of life, take steps to modify your personality. It's never to late to make important changes, but the time to start is *now!* The program described in the following sections is your key to success!

I see patients every day whose lifestyle habits put them at increased risk. Those who follow my advice and make the effort to change never regret it. One patient, CJE, is a good example of the success that can be achieved by following my risk-reducing plan. CJE first came to the Foundation for Study of Exercise, Stress and the Heart in 1978 for an evaluation of his health status and risk of disease development. He was 44 years old and 40 pounds (25%) overweight. Walking up hills left him out of breath, with his heart pounding heavily. His health risks were appalling; he scored at high risk on the risk-factor test with the odds favoring development of a serious health impairment.

After testing him, we discovered why CJE was at such high risk. He had smoked 1-1/2 packs of cigarettes a day for 20 years, drank four to six cocktails or glasses of wine every day, and used tranquilizers frequently to control headaches, tension and frustrations. He regularly used laxatives to overcome constipation and downed sleeping pills almost nightly. He was tense from morning to night, putting strain on his relationship with his wife and children because he rarely had time to enjoy a relaxed, pleasant time with them.

CJE's eating habits were a major cause for his overweight, constipation, insomnia and health risks. He had only a Danish and coffee for breakfast and drank more coffee later in the morning. Several times a week he took business associates out to a large lunch, eating a full-course meal and drinking martinis or wine. If he didn't have a business lunch, he'd have a "diet" lunch of a roast-beef sandwich or a cheeseburger.

When he walked around town after work or during the business day, he was often tempted to grab an ice-cream cone, hot dog or slice of pizza. To "relax" when he got home, he drank a martini or double scotch. More scotch accompanied a dinner of steak, lamb chops or roast beef. He rarely skipped dessert of ice cream, pie or cake, and the meal ended with coffee and often an after-dinner cordial. For a bedtime snack, he ate more dessert. If he brought work home in the evenings, he drank coffee to stay alert, then tried a shot of brandy or a sleeping pill to help himself get to sleep.

Though his health risks were high, he had a good family history because his mother and father were in their 70s and in good health. They were free from heart disease, high blood pressure, diabetes and cancer.

The chart below shows what baseline studies done at CJE's first visited reveal about his health risks.

CJE's FIRST VISIT

Age:	44
Height:	5' 10''
Weight:	207 pounds
Blood pressure:	150/100
Total cholesterol:	282mg/dl
HDL cholesterol:	34mg/dl
Triglycerides:	235mg/dl
Fasting glucose:	134mg/dl
2-hour glucose:	154mg/dl
Pulmonary vital capacity	60% of predicted
Cardiac exercise test	Poor performance for his age, as measured by oxygen consumption and the amount of exercise he was able to do before becoming short of breath and lightheaded.

When CJE learned how serious his risks were, he became committed to doing whatever it took to reduce them. He was serious about wanting to improve his health status and improve the quality of his relationship with his wife and children. He recognized he had a hyperreactive personality. He knew he had poor control of his eating, drinking and smoking habits and should get more exercise.

I arranged for CJE to consult a psychotherapist to help him sort out his goals and prioritize how to spend his time and energy. He made a series of visits and gained a new perspective on dealing with his job and family.

At the Foundation for Study of Exercise, Stress and the Heart, he was taught how to change his eating habits. Over a 6-month period, he gradually learned to avoid foods that were bad for him and to replace them with healthier choices.

He took time for a proper high-fiber breakfast in the morning and didn't need to rely on laxatives. Instead of a business lunch, he took colleagues on a long, brisk walk. He found business associates were glad not to have a formal meal and enjoyed a "business walk" instead of lunch. On other days, CJE ate a light lunch—a salad of salmon, lettuce and tomato. After lunch, rather than being half-asleep and devoid of self-control to resist late afternoon snacks, he found he was more alert and didn't need to work at home during the evenings to get his work done.

For dinner his wife now prepares a salad and two fresh vegetables every night. Rather than beef, she serves chicken and fish 5 times a week. Water accompanies every meal, and there is no bread or butter on the table to tempt CJE. He has learned to eat slowly and not take second portions. For dessert, he enjoys fruit and occasionally cheese. He stays out of the kitchen after dinner—except to help his wife and talk with her—and doesn't drink coffee or alcohol at the end of the meal or during the evening.

As for alcohol, it was easy to reduce his consumption once he realized how much better he felt when he cut it out. Now he doesn't drink at lunchtime. He drinks in the evenings only 5 days a week, drinking either three glasses of wine or two scotch and sodas (a total of 3 ounces of scotch) before and during the meal.

For exercise, CJE joined a club and learned to play squash. He also swims, does calisthenics and rides the exercycle. On weekends, he plays tennis, bicycles and hikes with his wife and children. Regular exercise has helped him lose weight and get his body in good physical condition.

It took 3 months of attending a quit-smoking course, but he finally stopped smoking completely and has not smoked since.

The psychotherapist helped CJE learn not to overreact to tension and stress and to take things in stride. Now he seldom needs Valium or a drink to calm him on difficult days. He doesn't need sleeping pills or a night-cap any more.

CJE is a changed man. His entire outlook is better. He smiles more and has a happier, more satisfying relationship with his wife and family. He is more confident and productive at his job. He is pleased with his appearance and vigor. He enjoys a sense of "well-being" and of being in control of his health and lifestyle.

His risk factors are greatly reduced. Three years after he first came to me, he scored at low risk on the risk-factor test, and his annual exam revealed remarkable changes for the better. See the chart on the following page.

After following my risk-reduction plan, CJE is a healthier, happier man today. By improving your lifestyle, you can significantly lower your risk. All you need to do is put into practice the nutrition and exercise plans that follow.

The diseases that strike down millions in the prime of their lives *don't* have to happen to you. Heart disease, stroke, cancer, diabetes and osteoporosis all depend largely on your lifestyle. You can significantly reduce your risk and protect your health by changing your diet and exercise habits, controlling your reaction to stress and making healthy lifestyle choices.

CJE's RISK REDUCTION

TEST	INITIAL VISIT	3 YEARS LATER	COMMENTS
Weight	207	171	From 25% overweight to normal
Blood pressure	150/100	135/80	Hypertension to normal
HDL-cholesterol	34mg/dl	48mg/dl	From risky to good
HDL/cholesterol ratio	8	4.5	From high risk to good
Triglyceride	235mg/dl	95mg/dl	From risky to good
Fasting glucose	134	94	From borderline diabetic to normal
2-hour glucose	154	105	From borderline diabetic to normal
Pulmonary function	60%	90%	From poor to normal
Cardiac stress test	30ml oxygen	48ml oxygen	From poor to good
RISK-ANALYSIS SCORE	High risk	Low risk	From high risk to low risk

15.

THE RISK-REDUCING NUTRITION PLAN

*TAKE THIS TEST TO MEASURE YOUR
NUTRITIONAL RISKS*

What you eat and in what amounts are two of the most important factors in determining your health. This test measures how nutritious your diet is. Circle the score for each characteristic that applies to you. Total the score as shown on page 189, then check your risk category on page 190.

1.   Which best describes your eating habits?

3. You usually eat generous portions at meals and snack between meals.

2. You eat large portions at meals but do not snack between meals.

1. You don't eat large portions at meals and rarely snack between meals, or you eat small portions at meals and have nutritious small snacks during the day.

2.   You salt your food:

3. Always, without tasting it.

2. Only during cooking, not at the table.

1. Neither during cooking nor at the table.

3. You eat packaged, prepared or restaurant foods:
   3. Regularly
   2. Occasionally
   1. Rarely

4. You eat bacon, sausage, hot dogs or cold cuts:
   3. Every day or almost every day
   2. About 3 times a week
   1. Rarely

5. You eat steak, hamburger or roast beef:
   3. 4 or more times a week
   2. 1 or 2 times a week
   1. Rarely

6. You eat chops or roasts of pork, beef or lamb:
   3. Several times a week
   2. About once a week
   1. Rarely

7. How many eggs, alone or as an ingredient in food, do you eat a week?
   3. 10 or more
   2. 5 or 6
   1. 2 or 3, or less

8. How often do you eat whole-grain or bran breakfast cereal?
   3. Rarely
   2. Several times a week
   1. Usually every day

9. How often do you eat whole-grain bread?
   3. Rarely
   2. Several times a week
   1. Every day

10. How often do you eat a rich dessert, such as ice cream, cake, pie or pastry?
    3. More than 3 times a week
    2. 2 or 3 times a week
    1. Rarely

11. How many servings of fruits or vegetables (not counting fruit juice) do you usually eat each day?
    3. 1 or none at all
    2. 2 or 3
    1. 4 or more

12. How often do you eat beans or legumes?
    3. Rarely
    2. 1 or 2 times a week
    1. Almost every day

13. You use butter rather than margarine:
    3. Always or almost always
    2. Sometimes
    1. Never use butter

14. You eat cheese (other than low-fat cottage cheese):
    3. 5 or more times a week
    2. About twice a week
    1. Rarely

15. You eat fish or shellfish:
    3. Less than once a week
    2. 1 or 2 times a week
    1. 3 or more times a week

16. You eat cabbage, cauliflower, broccoli or other cruciferous vegetables:
    3. 1 or 2 times a week
    2. 3 or 4 times a week
    1. Almost every day

17. You eat skim or low-fat dairy products:
    3. Rarely
    2. Once a day
    1. Several times a day

18. You eat whole-milk dairy products or cream:
    3. Every day
    2. 1 or 2 times a week
    1. Rarely

19. You eat skinless chicken or poultry (not fried):
    3. Rarely
    2. 1 or 2 times a week
    1. 3 or more times a week, instead of red meat

20. When you eat beef, you chose lean cuts and cut away as much fat as possible:
    3. Rarely
    2. Usually
    1. Always or almost always

21. For salads or cooking, you use polyunsaturated oils, such as corn, safflower or sunflower:
    3. Rarely
    2. Sometimes
    1. Usually

22. You use olive oil or peanut oil:
    3. Rarely
    2. Several times a week
    1. Every day or almost every day

23. You follow a fad or quick weight-loss diet:
    3. Every couple of months
    2. Less than once a year
    1. Never

24. You eat deep-fried foods:
    3. Almost every day
    2. 1 or 2 times a week
    1. Rarely

25. You eat orange or dark-green vegetables:
    3. 1 or less times a week
    2. 2 or 3 times a week
    1. Every day or almost every day

Calculating Your Score

Add up the number of 1s, 2s and 3s, fill them in below, and do the indicated calculations.

_____ (1s) x 1 = _____

_____ (2s) x 2 = _____

_____ (3s) x 3 = _____

Total Score _____

INTERPRETING YOUR SCORE

Check your total score below to see if your health and your life are at risk. You may be referred to the risk-reducing nutrition plan in this section.

25 to 32   **Low Risk**—You are following a nutritious diet that puts you at low risk of developing a life-threatening illness.

33 to 45   **Moderate Risk**—Your diet is good, and you are only at moderate risk of developing heart disease, cancer or diabetes due to diet-related effects.

46 to 60   **High Risk**—Your diet is adding to your risk of developing heart disease, cancer or diabetes. Follow the risk-reducing nutrition plan to lower your risk.

61 +   **Very High Risk**—Your diet may be putting you at very high risk of developing heart disease, cancer or diabetes. Begin the risk-reducing nutrition plan now to lower your risks and begin to help reverse the damage you have already done to your health.

TAKE THIS TEST TO MEASURE
HIDDEN CALORIES IN YOUR FOOD

This test measures hidden high-calorie foods in your diet that may contribute to your weight problem. Circle the score for each food you eat at least *once a week*. Check your total score on the opposite page to see if your health and your life are at risk.

+4   Danish pastry or donut for breakfast or midmorning snack
+6   Eggs and bacon for breakfast
+4   Salads (tuna, potato, egg) made with mayonnaise
+3   Creamy salad dressing
+6   Prime cut of steak or roast beef
+5   Beef pot pie
+4   Lamb chops
+5   Fried chicken
+4   Fast-food hamburger
+5   Spare ribs
+5   Hot dogs, salami, cold cuts
+3   Pizza
+4   French fries or fried onion rings

+4 Potato chips or similar snack foods
+3 Peanut butter
+4 Roasted nuts
+3 Dry-roasted nuts
+6 Cheese (other than low-fat cottage cheese)
+5 Ice cream
+5 Chocolate
+4 Beer
+3 Wine
+4 Mixed drink
+3 Straight liquor
+4 Sugared soft drinks or canned iced tea

INTERPRETING YOUR SCORE

To determine your score, add all scores. Check your total score below to see if your food choices are contributing to your overweight. You may be referred to the risk-reducing nutrition plan in this section or the risk-reducing exercise plan, page 226.

0 to 20 **Low Risk**—In addition to the calories in your diet, other factors are contributing to your weight problem. The risk-reducing exercise plan will help you lose weight.

21 to 29 **Moderate Risk**—Many foods you eat are high in hidden fat or sugar. By making better choices, you can begin to lose weight.

30+ **High Risk**—Your weight problem is due to excessive fat and sugar in your diet. Your choice of foods and the way they are prepared may be contributing to your weight problem. Learn what's in the food you eat, and follow the risk-reducing nutrition plan and risk-reducing exercise plan to achieve permanent weight loss.

The Risk-Reducing Nutrition Plan

Some diseases, such as arteriosclerosis, diabetes and certain cancers, may be in large part caused by your diet. If you follow my risk-reducing nutrition plan, you can lower your risk of these diseases. It's better to have followed a similar diet throughout your life, but if you start now, the benefits will accrue.

My nutrition plan is based on evidence gathered over the years from respected medical researchers and recommendations by the American Heart Association and the American Cancer Society. After considering evidence from research about how diet influences the diseases that strike us, I have devised a nutrition plan to help lower your risk of all these conditions. This lifetime plan for eating will help reduce your risk of cancer, heart disease, stroke, diabetes and osteoporosis.

This plan is designed for people who are at their desired weight and who do not need to lose weight. If you need to lose weight, follow the weight-loss diet that begins on page 204. Once you have lost the desired weight, switch to the risk-reducing nutrition plan to maintain your weight and your health.

OUR TYPICAL DIET

Our diet has always contained about 15% protein. Until the turn of the century, most of that protein came from vegetables, beans, wheat and other grains; these have little fat. Since 1900, the major source of dietary protein has come from animal products. Our typical diet today boasts an abundance of beef protein; beef could almost be considered a staple food.

Many of us love protein and erroneously believe we can't get too much of it and it isn't fattening. We are concerned about eating enough protein and mistakenly equate a 16-ounce sirloin-steak dinner with a healthy meal. The impact of this excessive amount of animal protein in our diets is clearcut. Consider the following:

- Countries where less meat is eaten and less fat ingested have a lower incidence of vascular disease, heart disease, colon cancer and breast cancer.
- A high-protein diet may cause loss of bone mass. When dietary-protein levels are too high, calcium is extracted from the bones and teeth and bound to protein in the body fluids, which leads to osteoporosis.
- Excess protein makes more demands on the kidneys and stresses them. In older people, whose kidneys function less efficiently, a high-protein diet can be harmful.
- Calories from excess protein are stored in the body primarily as body fat; protein can be fattening.

Until recently, athletes mistakenly equated beef with muscle power and ate large amounts of meat prior to competition. But this was really counterproductive because their bodies required a lot of extra water to wash out the excess nitrogen produced from digesting excessive amounts of protein. In metabolizing excess protein, cells can become dehydrated if you don't drink sufficient amounts of water (about 1 quart for every 1,000 calories of food a day); dehydration reduces energy and causes fatigue and collapse. Today, athletes eat less protein and more complex carbohydrates to provide more available energy and a better water balance.

But weight-conscious people have given complex carbohydrates an undeserved bad reputation. Complex carbohydrates, such as potatoes, bread and rice, are widely believed to be fattening, but that isn't true. These carbohydrates play an important role in a nutritious eating plan. Most starchy foods are of plant origin, so they contain little fat, but they do contain important vitamin and mineral nutrients and small amounts of protein. Ounce for ounce, pure carbohydrate has the same amount of calories as pure protein!

Carbohydrates are the mainstay of the risk-reducing nutrition plan. Nourishing vegetables supply the most nutrition for the lowest number of calories.

Fiber is important in my nutrition plan. It doesn't nourish your body, but evidence points to fiber as an important component in any nutritious diet. Fiber reduces the risk of bowel and breast cancers; it may play a role in heart-disease prevention because roughage slows the absorption of fat and cholesterol from the bowel. Fiber foods are filling and help control the appetite, also playing a role in weight reduction.

Fiber foods absorb water, leading to softer, bulkier stools that reduce pressure on the intestinal walls. Waste products move through the bowel at an increased rate; fats and potential carcinogens have less time in contact with the intestinal wall and less time to be absorbed, possibly reducing your risk of cancer. Because fiber needs to absorb water, you must increase the amount of water you drink daily if you eat a high-fiber diet. Failure to do so may result in constipation, which defeats the purpose of including fiber in your diet.

Whole grains are the best source of fiber, but fruits and vegetables are also excellent sources. All these foods are included in the risk-reducing nutrition plan.

Most of us eat too much fat. A high-fat diet carries with it the risk of coronary and vascular disease, increasing your chances of suffering a heart attack or stroke, and an increased danger of cancer. A high-fat diet may lead to obesity and its consequent complications. When we eat fatty meat and empty-calorie foods, we are consuming fat!

A diet high in saturated fat increases your body's production of cholesterol, which may increase your risk of coronary disease. For many people, an elevated serum-cholesterol level is the overriding factor in development of heart disease—for some people, diet is the deciding factor and for others it is a contributing factor. You should be conscious of keeping your cholesterol count as low as possible. It's vitally important to your health to limit dietary cholesterol and saturated fat to maintain the lowest serum-cholesterol and triglyceride levels possible.

193

Although a high-fat diet carries with it many risks for ill health, your body requires some dietary fat. It's vital to your well-being that at least 20% of your daily calories are from fat. I advise you to limit the type of fat in your diet to nutritious foods that contain some fat, such as poultry, seafood, low-fat dairy products, cereals, grains and vegetables, and small amounts of margarine and olive oil. Try to maintain an equal ratio between saturated, polyunsaturated and monounsaturated fats. Don't be misled into believing that because unsaturated fats do not have cholesterol they can be freely consumed. Excessive amounts of unsaturated fats are also linked to an increased incidence of breast, pancreatic and colon cancers.

THE BASICS OF THE RISK-REDUCING NUTRITION PLAN

The risk-reducing nutrition plan is a balanced plan based on what researchers know about the roles that fat, carbohydrate, protein, fiber, vitamins, minerals and alcohol play in the development of disease. Our typical diet derives 40% of its calories from fat, 15% from protein and 45% from carbohydrates. According to the latest research, this is too much fat and meat protein!

On the risk-reducing nutrition plan, you eat 20% fat, 15% protein and 65% carbohydrate—the 20-15-65 mix. The extra carbohydrates—complex sugars and starches—also provide you with protective vitamins and fiber.

Besides being too high in fat, our diet derives most of its fat from meat and dairy foods, which may contribute to heart disease and stroke. The American Heart Association advocates reducing fat to 30% and reducing the amount of saturated fat and cholesterol in the diet. Many people have heeded this and other advice concerning lifestyle and heart disease, and there has been a decrease in the number of deaths from heart attacks during the past 20 years. If this advice were followed on a more widespread scale, the occurrence of heart disease would probably drop even more dramatically.

Evidence is mounting as to the role dietary fat plays in cancer development. I believe 30% fat in the diet is still too high. In the risk-reducing nutrition plan, the percentage of fat is even lower, which should protect you from some kinds of cancer and heart disease.

We eat too much animal protein; most of this protein is loaded with extra fat calories. Your body only needs about 40 to 45 grams of protein a day—less than half of what most of us now eat! Most meat-loving Americans would find a diet containing only this small amount of protein too limited. On my nutrition plan, you can safely consume a little more protein than this because more of it is derived from vegetable sources. You can double the amount to 80 to 90 grams of low-fat protein—a healthy body can safely handle that amount. That's about 350 calories of protein a day.

A typical person eats 45% of his calories as carbohydrates. Many of those carbohydrate calories are derived from sugar rather than starches. Picture how large and heavy a 100-pound bag of cement is. Imagine the bag contained table sugar—that's how much sugar we consume in 1 year. In fact, many people eat much more than that! Sugar supplies little nourishment to your body. On the risk-reducing nutrition plan, you eat more starches and fibers, and fewer simple sugars.

My basic premise is to lower the amount of fat—saturated and unsaturated—and the amount of animal protein in your diet. The majority of calories come from complex carbohydrates—foods you might once have considered forbidden and fattening. But they are the best foods in your diet. Most vegetable foods contain some protein, so you'll be getting a large share of your daily protein from high-carbohydrate foods. See four sample menus, pages 201 and 202.

The nutrition plan provides you with sufficient calories and a balance of nutrients. You'll be able to eat delicious, satisfying foods and maintain your weight and health. You will eat more fiber from grains, beans, fruits and leafy vegetables. Fruits and vegetables containing cancer-preventing vitamins and other substances are included in every meal. Also included are calcium-rich foods to help prevent osteoporosis.

WHAT ARE THE FAT SOURCES?

With my nutrition plan, you lower your fat intake to 20% of your total daily calories. To protect yourself from heart disease and cancer, you eat equal portions of saturated, unsaturated and monounsaturated fats. Your protein sources will be mainly plant foods, poultry, fish and low-fat dairy products, so your saturated-fat level is lowered but not eliminated.

Meat will be the source of most of your saturated fat. To reduce the level of saturated fat, trim all visible fat from meat, and don't eat poultry skin. You need to know how to cook your food so it remains good for you. Steam or poach fish and shellfish, or bake or broil it with small amounts of fat. Use wine, herbs, lemon, lime and tomatoes for added flavor. Deep frying or creamy sauces counteract any health benefits.

To avoid excess fat calories, switch to low-fat dairy products. Choose skim milk and low-fat cottage cheese. Eliminate butter from your diet, and use soft-tub margarine to reduce saturated fat. Soft-tub margarines are best because they are less hydrogenated than solid bars and are more unsaturated.

Unsaturated oils include polyunsaturates and monounsaturates, which help lower serum-cholesterol levels. Excessive polyunsaturated fats may be involved in the development of some forms of cancer, so the risk-reducing nutrition plan helps balance your fat intake. Some people go overboard on polyunsaturates, to the exclusion of saturated fats, to avoid heart disease. By reducing your total fat intake and balancing the kinds of fat you eat, you're helping to protect yourself from heart disease and cancer.

Strive to balance the saturated, monounsaturated and polyunsaturated fats in your diet, so about 1/3 of the fat calories come from each source. This is the most nutritious mix. You can do this by using small quantities of unsaturated margarine and polyunsaturated oils, such as corn oil, safflower or sesame oil, and monounsaturated olive oil in preparing your food. If you use polyunsaturated oils in cooking, use olive oil in your salad. You get saturated fat from meat and poultry and from low-fat (not skim) dairy products.

The American Heart Association recommends that you keep your daily intake of cholesterol under 300mg. One egg yolk contains 275mg of cholesterol, so limiting eggs (or at least egg yolks) is a must. I advise my patients to eat no more than four eggs a week. If you eat two eggs one day, I suggest the rest of the day be cholesterol-free. This means no whole milk, butter, cheese, beef or organ meats.

Limit cheese, which is high in saturated fat, to the kinds with the lowest fat content. When preparing meat-free casseroles, choose low-fat mozzarella and ricotta cheese, and use low-fat cottage cheese. Organ meats, such as brain, liver and kidney, are full of fat and ready-made cholesterol—don't eat them at all!

WHAT ARE THE PROTEIN SOURCES?

The percentage of protein in the risk-reducing nutrition plan is 15%, which is close to what you are probably now eating, but the protein sources probably differ. You must change from a reliance on meat protein to include more plant and low-fat dairy protein. By doing this, the amount of fat in your diet is reduced, and you include more protective fiber, calcium and vitamins in your diet. You can probably eat 70 to 90 grams (280 to 360 calories) a day of protein if you are a woman eating 1,800 calories or a man eating 2,400 calories.

What foods should you eat to get protein in the most nourishing, tasty way? Let me give you an idea of how much protein is in some popular foods. A 3-ounce portion of steak, hamburger, pork roast, liver, leg of lamb or turkey each supply 22 to 26 grams of protein or about 100 calories of protein. These meats also give you fat calories! One-hundred fat calories come from the hamburger and as much as 250 fat calories come from the sirloin steak. Three ounces of shrimp, flounder or chicken breast provide the same number of protein calories as the meats listed, but with little or no fat. The message is clear—cut down on red meat, and eat more chicken and fish.

Evidence suggests meat fat contributes to the development of vascular heart disease, diabetes and cancer. Too much protein overloads your kidneys, causing waste products to be concentrated in your bloodstream, and depletes your bones of calcium. Reducing the amount of meat you eat and reducing the portions of total protein are essential if you want to reduce your risks of these conditions.

Eat meat, fish or poultry only once a day, and keep servings small—about 3 ounces for women and 4 ounces for men. One serving supplies about half of your allotment of protein calories—you still have another 100 calories of protein in your daily diet. You can get these easily—and nutritiously—from cereals, grains, low-fat dairy products and vegetables. For example, a serving of dried breakfast cereal supplies 25 to 30 calories of protein. When you add a cup of skim milk, you get another 35 calories of protein. Cottage cheese (low-fat) has 40 to 50 calories of protein; brown rice, 40 to 50; whole-wheat flour, 50; broccoli, Brussels sprouts, corn, peas and spinach all have about 20 to 25 calories of protein per serving. Half a cup of beans (lima, kidney, navy) provide 60 calories of protein, and soybeans have as much protein calories as 3 ounces of steak—between 90 and 110. See Appendix, which begins on page 237.

Eat beef, lamb or pork only once a week. Eat poultry or fish for the remaining six animal-protein-based meals. Include cold-water fish that contain protective omega-3 fatty acids in your diet several times a week. The fish that contain these protective fats include salmon, mackeral, bluefish, tuna, swordfish, sardines, mullet, herring, sablefish, trout, shad, butterfish and pompano. Shrimp, lobster and crab also contain some protective omega-3 fatty acids; the cholesterol they contain is about as much as in chicken, so they may be eaten in moderation. Clams, mussels, oysters and scallops, which are low in cholesterol, may be eaten freely.

This plan is probably a major departure from your customary diet, but our record on heart disease and cancer is certainly not enviable. Much of your protein requirement can be filled from carbohydrate foods, such as beans, legumes and grains, and low-fat milk and cheeses; these supply protein (and calcium) without saturated fat. When combined properly with each other or with small portions of meat or dairy products, vegetable protein can become complete.

WHAT ARE THE CARBOHYDRATE SOURCES?

By increasing the carbohydrate content of your diet to approximately 65%, you include more vegetables, fruits, pastas, cereals and grains. Start to think of these foods as the mainstay of your diet; between 1,200 and 1,600 calories, depending on your activity level and current weight, will be supplied by the carbohydrates you eat. Of this, the majority (about 90%) come from vegetables, fruits, beans, cereals, bread and pasta. Grains, breads and pastas in normal portions are not fattening unless covered with butter or cream sauces. Use pasta and grains as the basis for satisfying meatless meals. Choose whole-grain breads, such as oatmeal and whole-wheat, rather than white bread.

Every day, 100 to 150 calories can be used in the form of simple carbohydrates, which can come from alcohol, added sugar or an occasional treat, such as ice cream or cake. Keep in mind 1 teaspoon of sugar contains 16 calories—but in heavily sweetened foods, those calories add up. Most soft drinks contain 10 to 12 teaspoons of sugar in a 12-ounce can!

The risk-reducing nutrition plan drastically reduces the amount of unnecessary sugar in your daily diet. Your weight will benefit, your teeth will benefit and you'll reduce the chances of developing diabetes. You'll be getting your calories from healthier foods, so you'll also reduce your risks of cancer and heart disease.

Eat at least four servings of fruits and vegetables every day. I recommend six servings—two at each meal. Vegetables should be fresh or frozen, never canned; canned vegetables contain too much sodium and lose nutrients in the canning liquid. Choose fresh fruit in season or frozen fruit, without sugar. Choose whole, fresh fruits over fruit juice because your body derives better blood-sugar control from whole fruits, and it also gets added fiber.

WHAT ARE THE FIBER SOURCES?

My nutrition plan contains 25 to 30 grams of fiber from vegetable and grain sources. Drink at least 6 ounces of water with each meal to avoid constipation.

Many of the complex-carbohydrate sources that are the mainstay of the plan are high-fiber foods, so you don't have to make a special effort to include these. I usually recommend a breakfast of high-fiber cereal. Mix 1/4 to 1/2 cup of 100% bran with 3/4 to 1 cup of another whole-grain cereal, such as Shredded Wheat, corn flakes or wheat flakes.

The best sources of fiber are oatmeal, whole-grain bread, bran cereal, peas, beans, broccoli, Brussels sprouts, corn, cabbage, carrots, whole-wheat cereals, Shredded Wheat, Puffed Wheat, baked potatoes, apples, strawberries and raspberries. Other fruits and vegetables contain fiber but in smaller quantities. Any of these should help supply enough fiber when eaten along with high-fiber sources.

Although fiber is an important part of your nutrition plan, you can overdo it. Excess fiber can block iron and calcium absorption and remove vitamin B-12, folic acid and the fat-soluble vitamins. It can result in the accumulation of too much gas in the intestinal tract, causing flatulence and bloating. If you currently eat a low-fiber diet, add fiber to your diet gradually so your system can adjust without producing excess gas. Flatulence is usually a temporary condition that goes away when your digestive system adapts to the increased fiber. As always, a balance of good food is still the goal.

WHAT ARE THE VITAMIN AND MINERAL SOURCES?

The evidence for vitamin A (beta-carotene) and vitamin C as cancer preventives is very strong, though not conclusive. Vitamins A and C are important in building a strong immune system and are important components of the risk-reducing nutrition plan, which includes foods high in these vitamins in almost every meal.

You need vitamin C every day because it is a water-soluble vitamin that is excreted from the body. I suggest each meal include a fruit or vegetable high in vitamin C, such as an orange, grapefruit, lemon, strawberries, cantaloupe, green and red peppers, asparagus, broccoli or cabbage. This is important if you eat meat because vitamin C is needed to absorb iron. If you don't include the high-vitamin-C food at a meal, have it as a snack during the day.

Eat at least one generous serving of high-vitamin-A foods every day. These are generally the highly pigmented fruits and vegetables, such as carrots or cantaloupe. The deeper-orange or darker-green fruits and vegetables contain the most beta-carotene, which your body converts to vitamin A.

Compounds called *dithiolthione* are found in cabbage-family vegetables, and they seem to protect against cancer. The American Cancer Society advocates eating these vegetables frequently, so they are included in the nutrition plan. One serving a day of broccoli, cauliflower, Brussels sprouts, kohlrobi, cabbage or watercress is included. These vegetables are also good sources of fiber and vitamins A and C and are excellent risk-reducing foods.

WHAT ARE THE CALCIUM SOURCES?

Enough calcium—about 1,000mg—for an average adult is included in the foods you eat. Four 8-ounce servings of skim milk or the equivalent in low-fat cottage cheese or yogurt should be included in each day's menu to help reduce your risk of high blood pressure and osteoporosis. Dairy products also supply a significant portion of protein. Additional calcium comes from leafy green vegetables.

Teens and pregnant or lactating women should drink more milk to fulfill their greater calcium needs. Menopausal women may need a calcium supplement to give them the extra protection they need to prevent osteoporosis. The amount of additional calcium needed depends on age and other factors. A woman at risk of kidney stones should not take calcium supplements unless advised by her physician who knows her medical history. Before you begin taking calcium supplements, check with your doctor.

HOW TO PREPARE YOUR FOOD

Try to use as little fat as possible when preparing food. Switch from fried vegetables to steamed, from fried chicken or fish to poached. For added flavor, cook fish and poultry in wine and herbs; add lemon juice or tomatoes for variety. Remove all visible fat from meats. Use a non-stick frying pan and sauté vegetables or meats in a small amount of olive or sesame oil for a delicious flavor without excess fat calories.

Make your own salad dressing from vinegar and olive oil instead of using prepared dressings or those based on sour cream. Rather than the usual 2 tablespoons of oil to 1 tablespoon of vinegar, use a 1:1 ratio. Select a fragrant specialty vinegar found at gourmet food stores. Many of these vinegars taste sweeter and can be used in larger quantities than you would typically use cider vinegar. Don't salt your salad dressing;

199

use pepper, dry mustard, fresh dill, parsley or lemon juice for flavor.

Avoid the salt shaker—keep it off the table. Salt foods only lightly when cooking. If you have high blood pressure, don't salt at all. If you are "addicted" to salt, it will be difficult to cut down—do so gradually. Over several weeks, you should be able to wean your family from excess salt; what once tasted fine to you will taste surprisingly and unpleasantly salty.

You probably can't make all these changes overnight, but begin by setting long-term, reasonable goals. Your ultimate goal may be to reduce your meat protein consumption and your fat intake by half the amounts you probably eat now. Your new diet, filled with carbohydrates, will still be satisfying. In fact, it will "fill" you up more easily, and you'll feel satisfied longer. Try it. There's a great variety of delicious carbohydrate foods to choose from that are better for you than animal protein because of their low-fat content and their fiber content. You'll probably enjoy them or learn to enjoy them just as much.

WHAT YOU DRINK IS IMPORTANT

The best thing you can drink is water. Drink plenty of it to assure the fiber you eat is processed correctly. Drink only one or two cups of coffee a day to reduce the possible risks of pancreatic cancer, raising serum-cholesterol levels and hyperstimulation of the brain and heart. Alcohol consumption must be kept at or below moderate levels—3 ounces (two shots) of hard liquor or two 12-ounce glasses of beer or two 5-ounce glasses of wine a day, no more than 5 days a week.

Keep regular soft drinks to a minimum; they provide too much sugar, which rushes into your bloodstream, upsetting your blood-sugar control mechanisms. Avoid diet drinks for several reasons. Sugar substitutes are suspected low-level carcinogens and active cancer promoters (enhancing growth of tumors already present). Research by Dr. Richard Wurtman at MIT indicates aspartame may affect the brain, causing you to crave more sweets. This defeats the purpose of a diet drink! Soft drinks also contain large amounts of phosphorous, which may deplete the calcium in your system.

SAMPLE MENUS

On the next two pages are four sample menus designed for men and women who are physically active and who do not need to lose weight. For women, daily menus contain about 2,000 calories. For men, they contain about 2,200 calories. Both plans average 20% fat, 15% protein and 65% carbohydrate. The foods in each day's menu also contain calcium, fiber, vitamin A, vitamin C and dithiolthiones.

SAMPLE MENUS

#1	Cal	Fat (g)	Protein (g)	Carb (g)
Breakfast				
1 medium orange	65	0.1	1.4	16.3
1/3 c. 100% bran	170	2.8	7	41.4
1/2 c. whole-grain corn flakes	55	0.5	1	11.7
10 halves dried apricots	83	0.2	1.3	21.6
8 oz. 1% low-fat milk	102	2.6	4.2	11.7
1 c. coffee or tea	3			0.5
Subtotal	*478*	*6.2*	*14.9*	*103.2*
Lunch				
Pear & cottage cheese salad				
made of:				
Pear	98	0.7	0.7	25.1
1 c. cottage cheese	217	9.5	26.2	5.6
4 whole-wheat breadsticks	96	1.2		17.2
1 small piece gingerbread	267	12.9	3	35
with 1 T. applesauce	13	0.1	0.1	3.1
Subtotal	*691*	*24.4*	*30*	*86*
Dinner				
3 oz. sole filet, baked in 3-1/2 oz.	80	0.5	14.9	0.6
herbed white-wine sauce	80		0.2	3.4
3 small parslied potatoes	120	0.1	3.1	25.6
1 c. Brussels sprouts	36	0.4	4.2	6.4
1/2 acorn squash	86	0.2	3	21.8
1 c. coleslaw	24	0.2	1.3	5.4
with 1 T. dressing	31	3.4	0.1	
1 small slice pound cake	123	5.6	1.9	16.4
with 1/2 c. sliced strawberries	45	0.6	0.9	10.5
Subtotal	*625*	*11*	*29.6*	*90.1*
Snack				
8 oz. 1% low-fat milk	102	2.6	8	11.9
1 medium banana	105	0.6	1.2	26.7
2 graham-cracker squares	60	1.5	1	10.8
Subtotal	*267*	*4.7*	*10.2*	*49.4*
Total for women	**2061**	**46.3**	**84.7**	**328.7**
Percentage for women		20.4	16.6	64.36
Men extra				
1 small parslied potato	40		1	8.5
1/3 c. fresh grapes	94	0.1	0.6	25.2
Subtotal	*134*	*.1*	*1.6*	*33.7*
Total for men	**2195**	**46.4**	**86.3**	**362.4**
Percentage for men		19.2	15.9	66.59

#2	Cal	Fat (g)	Protein (g)	Carb (g)
Breakfast				
1 c. blueberries	82	0.6	1	20.5
1-1/2 oz. Shredded Wheat	166	0.6	5.2	37.6
4 oz. 1% low-fat milk	51	1.3	4	5.8
1/2 whole-wheat bagel	59	1.1	2.3	10.9
1 t. soft margarine	17	1.9		
1 c. coffee or tea	3			0.5
Subtotal	*378*	*5.5*	*12.5*	*75.3*
Lunch				
Fresh fruit salad made of:				
1/2 c. apple	81	0.5	0.3	21.1
1/2 c. pineapple	39	0.3	0.3	9.6
1/2 c. peaches	37	0.1	0.6	9.7
1/2 c. strawberries	23	0.3	0.5	5.3
3/4 c. low-fat, plain yogurt	108	2.7	9	12
1 whole-wheat breadstick	24	0.3		4.3
3/4 c. raspberry sherbet	177		2.1	43.2
Subtotal	*489*	*4.2*	*12.8*	*105.2*
Dinner				
6 oz. red wine	140		0.4	**5**
2 lamb loin chops, trimmed	205	10.9	24.9	
1 large potato, baked	139	0.2	3.9	31.7
2 t. soft margarine	34	3.8		
2/3 c. steamed carrots	31	0.2	0.9	7.1
3/4 c. steamed peas	84	0.4	6.3	14.4
Salad made of:				
1 medium orange	65	0.1	1.4	16.3
1 T. onion	4		0.2	0.9
10 shredded radishes	17	0.1	1	3.6
1 T. oil & vinegar dressing	69	7.5		1.2
3/4 c. vanilla ice milk	184	5.6	5.2	29
Subtotal	*972*	*28.8*	*44.2*	*109.2*
Snack				
1 medium apple	81	0.5	0.3	21.1
1 garlic breadstick	24	0.3		4.3
8 oz. 1% low-fat milk	102	2.6	8	11.7
Subtotal	*207*	*3.4*	*8.3*	*37.1*
Total for women	**2046**	**41.9**	**77.8**	**326.8**
Percentage for women		18.4	15.2	63.89
Men extra				
1 piece cornbread	198	7.3	4.1	28.7
Subtotal	*198*	*7.3*	*4.1*	*28.7*
Total for men	**2244**	**49.2**	**81.9**	**355.5**
Percentage for men		19.7	14.6	63.37

SAMPLE MENUS

#3	Cal	Fat (g)	Protein (g)	Carb (g)
Breakfast				
1 peach	37	0.1	0.6	9.7
1/3 c. 100% bran	170	2.8	7	41.4
1/2 c. puffed wheat	26	0.1	1.1	5.4
8 oz. 1% low-fat milk	102	2.6	8	11.7
1/2 whole-wheat bagel	59	1.1	2.3	10.9
1 t. soft margarine	17	1.9		
1 c. coffee or tea	3			0.5
Subtotal	*414*	*8.6*	*19*	*79.6*
Lunch				
1-1/2 c. vegetarian chili made of:				
1 c. tomatoes	78	0.2	1.6	11
1/2 c. kidney beans	100	0.4	7.7	23.4
1 T. green bell pepper	11		0.6	2.4
1 T. onion	29		1.2	6.5
6 Ritz crackers	104	2.9	0.6	5.5
3/4 c. pineapple pudding				
(instant) made with whole milk	258	6.4	6	45.6
1/3 c. fresh grapes	94	0.1	0.6	25.2
Subtotal	*674*	*10*	*18.3*	*119.6*
Dinner				
4 oz. sesame chicken cutlet				
(breaded with 1 t. flour, 1 T.				
sesame seeds)	166	5.3	27.8	0.4
3/4 c. wild rice pilaf	147	1.8	3.2	25
1 c. steamed green beans	31	0.2	2	6.8
Tossed green salad made of:				
1 c. salad greens	13	0.1	0.9	2.9
10 radishes	17	0.1	1	3.6
1 T. olive oil & vinegar dressing	69	7.5		0.6
1 medium corn muffin	141	4.5	3.2	21.6
2 t. soft margarine	34	3.8		
1-1/4 c. fresh fruit compote				
made of:				
1/2 c. strawberries	23	0.3	0.5	5.2
1/4 c. blueberries	21	0.1	0.2	5.1
1/2 banana	52	0.3	0.6	13.3
1/4 c. lemon juice	16	0	0.4	5.2
1/2 t. cinnamon	3			0.9
Subtotal	*733*	*24*	*39.8*	*90.6*
Snack				
1 medium apple	81	0.5	0.3	21.1
8 oz. 1% low-fat milk	102	2.6	8	11.7
Subtotal	*183*	*3.1*	*8.3*	*32.8*
Total for women	2004	45.7	85.4	322.6
Percentage for women		20.7	17.2	64.97
Men extra				
1/4 c. pineapple pudding	88	2.2	2	15.9
1/4 c. wild rice pilaf	49	0.2	0.5	4.5
1/2 c. fruit compote	100	0.4	1.1	18.7
Subtotal	*237*	*2.8*	*3.6*	*39.1*
Total for men	2241	48.5	89	361.7
Percentage for men		19.6	16.0	65.08

#4	Cal	Fat (g)	Protein (g)	Carb (g)
Breakfast				
1-1/2 c. cantaloupe chunks	78	0.6	1.9	17.4
1 c. rice cereal	112	0.2	1.9	24.8
1 c. whole-grain cornflakes	55	0.1	1	11.7
1 t. sugar	16			2
1 banana	105	0.6	1.2	26.7
4 oz. 1% low-fat milk	51	1.3	4	5.8
1 c. coffee or tea	3			0.5
Subtotal	*420*	*2.8*	*10*	*88.9*
Lunch				
1 oz. Swiss cheese	107	7.8	8.1	1
2 slices cracked-wheat bread	122	1.8	4.6	25
1 t. mustard	3	0.2	0.2	0.3
3/4 c. carrot sticks	42	0.2	1.1	9.7
1 c. tossed green salad	13	0.1	0.9	2.9
1 T. cooked dressing	25	1.5		0.6
1 apple, baked	91	0.6	0.5	23.2
with 1 T. apple butter	37	0.2	0.1	9.1
Subtotal	*440*	*12.4*	*15.5*	*71.8*
Dinner				
Shrimp & broccoli stir fry,				
made with:				
1 c. shrimp	90	0.8	18.8	1.5
1 T. onion & garlic	13		0.2	0.9
1 c. chicken broth	37	1.4	1.3	0.9
1 T. lemon juice	4		0.1	1.3
2 T. cornstarch	70			16.6
1 c. broccoli	27	0.2	2.9	4.9
2 t. vegetable oil	80	6.4		
1 c. rice, cooked	164	0.2	3	36.3
2 baking-powder biscuits	182	6.2	4	26.6
1 t. soft margarine	17	1.9		
1 c. low-fat plain yogurt	144	3.5	11.9	16
1 c. fresh blueberries	82	0.1	0.6	20.5
Subtotal	*910*	*20.7*	*42.8*	*125.5*
Snack				
8 oz. 1% low-fat milk	102	2.6	8	11.7
1 medium tangelo	39	0.1	0.5	9.2
Subtotal	*141*	*2.7*	*8.5*	*20.9*
Total for women	1911	38.6	76.8	307.1
Percentage for women		18.2	16.1	64.28
Men extra				
1 medium pear	98	0.7	0.7	25.1
1 oz. Swiss cheese	107	7.8	8.1	1
1/3 c. rice, cooked	55	0.1	0.1	12.1
3 graham-cracker squares	90	2.2	1.5	16.2
Subtotal	*350*	*10.8*	*10.4*	*54.4*
Total for men	2261	49.4	87.2	361.5
Percentage for men		19.7	15.4	63.95

WHAT ARE THE MAJOR DIETARY CHANGES?

The major dietary change you'll have to make is to reduce the amount of meat, especially beef, that you probably eat. At the same time, you must increase your consumption of complex carbohydrates.

Your body needs only 40 to 45 grams of protein a day, but we typically eat 80 to 100 grams daily. Any extra protein you eat is stored in your body as fat!

Excess animal protein is loaded with excess dietary fat. Too much of this protein results in less bowel bulk, which may lead to diverticulitis and colon cancer. Much of your daily protein needs can be supplied from the complex carbohydrates you eat.

With my nutrition plan, you must eliminate or drastically reduce certain foods in your diet and increase other foods. The following rules summarize the basic concepts of the diet:

- Eat no more than 3 or 4 eggs a week, alone or as ingredients in prepared foods.
- Eat meat, poultry or fish only once a day.
- Reduce red-meat consumption to no more than one 3- to 4-ounce serving a week.
- Don't eat poultry skin.
- Eat bacon, hot dogs, salami and other nitrite- or nitrate-containing processed meats no more than once a month.
- Eat cold-water fish containing omega-3 fatty acids at least twice a week.
- Eat three servings a day of skim or low-fat dairy products.
- Take calcium supplements under your doctor's supervision if you are female.
- Eat whole-grain breads and cereals.
- Eat a high-vitamin-C fruit or vegetable at every meal.
- Eat a high-vitamin-A fruit or vegetable at least once a day.
- Eat a cabbage-family vegetable once a day.
- Choose whole fruits over fruit juice.
- Eat only fresh or frozen vegetables.
- Avoid processed and packaged food and empty-calorie foods.
- Don't add salt to food at the table; use salt sparingly while cooking.
- Use margarine (soft tub is best) instead of butter.
- Use olive oil for salads.
- Use polyunsaturated oil for cooking.
- Don't eat rich desserts more than once a week.
- Drink no more than 2 cups of coffee (caffeinated or decaffeinated) a day.
- Don't drink soft drinks on a regular basis, including diet soda.
- Consume no more than 3 ounces (two shots) of hard liquor or two 12-ounce glasses of beer or two 5-ounce glasses of wine a day, no more than 5 days a week.

16.

LOSE WEIGHT PERMANENTLY, WITHOUT RISK

If you're overweight, you probably need to lose weight so you'll feel better and look better. You'll also protect your health. But how can you diet safely, without risk? If you've read the section on fad diets, which begins on page 170, you know quick-weight-loss diets don't work for long-term weight loss. So how can you keep off those extra pounds permanently? How can you lose weight safely, without risking your health?

In this section, I give you answers to these important questions. You can shed extra fat safely and permanently through a combination of good nutrition, calorie counting and exercise. Discard the fad diets forever, and follow my recommendations, which are based on sound medical advice.

WHAT IS YOUR IDEAL WEIGHT?

The concept of ideal weight is controversial. No number represents a "best weight" for any individual. Physicians and insurance companies have traditionally relied on a weight table devised by the Metropolitan Life Insurance Co. as a measure of ideal weight. The table is based on statistics for longevity of various weights for men and women of small, medium and heavy builds. Several years ago, this table was updated, and ideal weights were *increased,* causing great debate that still rages on today.

It has been my experience that a person can be 10 pounds above or 10 pounds below the weight on the insurance chart and still be healthy. All the chart represents is a *range* of weight for healthy people. The closer you stay to that range, while healthy, the better you will function and feel. Other factors, such as how much you exercise and what you eat, must also be considered.

Rather than using the Metropolitan chart, I use a formula to calculate the ideal weight of my patients. You can also use this to gauge your ideal weight range.

If you're a man, start with a weight of 106 pounds, and add 6 pounds for every inch of your height over 5 feet. This is your ideal weight if you have a medium build. Add 10% of this weight to the figure if you have a muscular, heavy-boned build. Subtract 10% if you have a slender build.

For a man 5' 10" tall:

106 pounds + (6 pounds x 10) = 166 pounds for medium build

166 pounds − 16.6 pounds = about 150 pounds for a slim build

166 pounds + 16.6 pounds = about 182 pounds for a heavy build

Weight range: 150 to 182 pounds

If you are a woman, start with a weight of 100 pounds, and add 5 pounds for every inch of your height over 5 feet. This is your ideal weight if you have a medium build. Add 10% of this weight to the figure if you have a heavy-boned build. Subtract 10% if you have a slender build.

For a woman 5' 4" tall:

100 pounds + (5 pounds x 4) = 120 pounds for medium build

120 pounds − 12 pounds = 108 pounds for slim build

120 pounds + 12 pounds = 132 pounds for a heavy build

Weight range: 108 to 132 pounds

From these formulas you can see your body build is significant in determining how much you ought to weigh. If you fall into the high range for a given height category, don't label yourself big-boned—look in the mirror. You might also check in various books to determine what size frame you have; often the size of your wrist or an elbow-width measurement is used as a determinant. You aren't doing yourself any favors by rationalizing excess pounds.

You may be concerned about whether or not you need to lose weight. If you're between 10 and 15 pounds overweight, according to the weight tables, you might ask yourself whether you should shed those extra pounds. How much weight do you actually need to lose?

These are important concerns. But even if you are a few pounds above the recommended weight for your height and build, it may not be advisable for you to lose any weight. The first consideration is whether or not you are in good health. If you have high blood pressure, heart trouble, diabetes, kidney disease, arthritis or other serious diseases and are overweight, shed those extra pounds! If not, statistically you have no greater probability of developing disease or dying earlier by being within 10 to 15% of your ideal weight.

Excess overweight, or obesity, is a risk factor in many diseases. You may not like to characterize yourself as obese, but if you are more than 20% above your ideal weight, you are clinically obese. Such excessive body weight puts you at risk of sudden death, angina pectoris, heart failure, high blood pressure and some forms of cancer. Although data indicates obesity is not one of the major risk factors of cardiovascular disease, it is still important, especially for those under age 50 and for those who have other risk factors, such as smoking.

For excessively overweight people, statistics show an increased incidence of heart disease and sudden death because of cardiac disease. Obese men also have a 20% decrease in life expectancy. Obese women have a 10% decrease. This shortening of life is generally due to complications of hypertension, diabetes and gallbladder disease.

If you are sedentary and overeat regularly, you may weigh above the weight that is healthy for you. If you are morbidly obese, meaning you are 50% or more over your ideal weight, the risk of developing heart disease, cancer, diabetes or other major illnesses is much greater than if you were at a normal weight. Conversely, if you have heart disease or diabetes and are at least 15 to 20% overweight, the chances of helping yourself improve your health or even cure the condition are greatly enhanced by bringing you closer to the normal-weight range.

If you are presently in good health, your future health doesn't depend on your shedding an extra 10 pounds. But each of us is a potential candidate for some kind of cardiovascular disease sooner or later, so losing the extra weight won't hurt unless you crash diet.

If you are at what you consider your ideal weight and usually maintain that weight, don't panic if you gain a few pounds. You can lose the extra weight by watching your calories for a few weeks until you get your body back to the weight you want. When you are close to your ideal weight, adjust your food intake.

Some overweight people who want to lose weight for appearance's sake go on a crash diet several times a year. They lose weight only to gain it back again. This is called *yo-yoing,* and it is worse for your health than staying a few steady pounds above your ideal weight because it forces your body to constantly readjust its metabolism. It also lowers your self-esteem when you attempt to diet and fail.

If your weight is 10 to 15% above what it should be, don't start a diet merely to abandon it. It's more important to maintain a well-balanced diet than it is to lose excess pounds.

HOW MANY CALORIES DO YOU NEED?

It is a scientific fact that all the calories you eat are used to provide your body with energy, or they are stored as body fat. One pound of body fat equals 3,500 calories. That means if most people eat 500 calories more than they burn up through exercise or metabolism every day for 1 week, they would gain 1 pound of body fat. Those 500 calories could easily come from a piece of chocolate cake, several beers or a generous sirloin steak.

Everyone's metabolism is unique. You burn up a given number of calories just to maintain your weight and to carry out your body's everyday chemical reactions. This is called your *basal metabolic rate (BMR),* which is the number of calories your body needs every day to maintain itself if you were doing nothing more than lying flat on your back. Add to this the number of calories your body needs for the energy you expend through your daily activities—walking, working, carrying groceries, running for the subway—and you get the number of calories you expend every day.

Your body is inclined to seek the most "fuel efficient" metabolism and always attempts to consume less energy. As you grow older, your BMR slows down, requiring less energy. With middle age, many of us become more sedentary, and as a result, our bodies require fewer calories.

To maintain your ideal weight in this situation, you must eat less. This is unfortunate for those who like to eat, and it means more of the calories we eat must represent nutritious foods—there is less leeway for empty calories. The food you eat must count toward supplying your body with the nutrients it needs to function at its peak.

It's possible to overcome a slowdown in basal metabolic rate and not grow wider as you grow older. You can increase your amount of exercise so you burn more calories. If you don't exercise more, you must reduce your caloric intake to balance your lower metabolic rate. Many overweight people haven't adjusted their diets to this point of balance.

A generous diet for a sedentary person provides about 2,000 calories a day. Most of us rarely use that many calories unless we are athletes, farmers or construction workers. Anything in excess of the amount your metabolism uses results in weight gain unless it is burned off.

It's easy to consume 2,000 calories without realizing it. If you drink two scotch and sodas, you consume about 400 calories. That leaves only 1,600 for the rest of the day's food. One meal in a restaurant with drinks, appetizers, dressings, sauces and dessert can easily be 2,000 calories. Unless you run or do other strenuous exercise, it's difficult to maintain a caloric balance and keep your weight steady.

Everyone is entitled to some empty calories occasionally, sometimes just for self-gratification. For those who manage to maintain their weight at acceptable levels—within 15% or so of suggested weight—an occasional departure from a diet is permissible. But sooner or later, you'll have to make up for it by exercising or restricting your calories if you don't want to gain weight.

To begin to understand how you can lose weight safely and permanently, you need to understand exactly how many calories you need and how many you are currently consuming. The formula on the following page indicates the approximate number of calories you actually burn daily, depending on your weight and activity level. This may vary between individuals because of age and differences in basal metabolic rate, but it is a useful approximation. If you like to eat, you may find the number of calories your body burns is fewer than you usually consume, and that's the crux of your weight problem.

Determine your activity level from the chart below. Ten is for the most sedentary people—a man who works at a desk job, comes home and sits down in front of the TV every night, doing little more than mowing the lawn once a week and walking the dog around the block. (Most of us have an activity level of 14 or less.)

10 to 12: Minimal or no physical activity. A sedentary desk job, little or no vigorous exercise.
13 to 15: Relatively inactive job but a fairly regular physical exercise program 3 to 5 times a week.
16 to 18: Heavy activity or strenuous physical job, equally active non-working hours (farmers, construction workers, professional athletes).

After you have determined your activity level, multiply that number by your present weight.

Example: 150-pound man with an activity level of 13:

150 pounds x 13 = 1,950 calories

This individual burns about 1,950 calories a day. Even if he were engaging in strenuous activity, he would use only about 2,500 calories a day.

Looking at the caloric values of ordinary foods—the ones on the risk-reducing nutrition plan—you can see there isn't much room for extras, such as high-calorie junk foods or rich desserts.

YOU CAN LOSE WEIGHT WITHOUT RISK

My permanent-weight-loss diet is based on the generally accepted theory that for most people 1 pound of body fat represents 3,500 calories. If each day for 1 week you ate 500 calories *more* than your body burned up through its metabolism, at the end of that week you would probably have gained 1 pound. Conversely, to lose 1 pound in a week, you would probably need a total deficit of 3,500 calories.

Many dieters set unrealistic goals for themselves. If you expect to lose 5 pounds in 1 week—as many fad diets promise—that's equal to a weekly calorie reduction of 17,500 calories. This is practically impossible to do because the average person of normal weight requires 2,000 calories a day (14,000 calories a week) to maintain his weight. You'd have to fast, and then some, to lose 5 pounds of body fat.

The reason you may be able to lose 5 pounds during the first week on a quick-weight-loss diet is you really lose *water* not body fat. The water-weight loss is not permanent and may be hazardous to your health.

My permanent-weight-loss diet doesn't promise quick weight loss, but it does promise you'll lose weight slowly and steadily, and you'll keep those pounds off. The first step is to set a realistic goal for yourself. If you need to lose 20 pounds, plan on 4 to 6 months to do so. Any more rapid weight loss means you'll be depriving your body of necessary nutrients. You may feel so deprived of food you quit the diet because you can't stand suffering any longer.

Set a long-range goal so you have time to make permanent changes in your eating habits. Don't immediately shoot for your ideal weight. Aim for something you think you can achieve—maybe 1 pound a week. Setting an unrealistic goal is another way to defeat a diet and prove you don't want to lose weight. Settle on something attainable.

If you currently consume 2,100 calories a day (14,700 calories a week), you need to cut back to 1,600 calories a day. You can do this by eating less or exercising more to burn some or all of the extra calories. Beginning on page 226, I describe the best kinds of exercise and tell you how to do it safely. Read the section carefully, and use the information to select the amount and kind of exercise to suit your needs.

You can design a customized weight-loss diet for yourself. Take your present weight, and use the formula on the opposite page to calculate how many calories you are eating each day to maintain your present state of overweight. Determine what your ideal weight is. Plug this number into the formula to see how many calories you would be eating if you were at your *ideal weight*. Subtract the smaller number of calories from the larger number to see how many fewer calories a day you would need to reach your desired weight.

For this example, let's use a 175-pound man who is sedentary, whose ideal weight is 155 pounds, with an activity level of 12.

Calories consuming to maintain weight:
175 pounds x 12 = 2,100 calories
Calories needed to maintain present weight with increased activity level:
175 pounds x 15 = 2,625
Calories needed to maintain ideal weight at present activity level:
155 pounds x 12 = 1,860 calories
Calories needed to maintain ideal weight with increased activity:
155 pounds x 15 = 2,325 calories

From these calculations, you can see if this overweight person increased his activity level significantly and was burning up more than 500 calories a day exercising, he would lose about 1 pound a week without changing his eating habits.

If he reduced his caloric intake to the amount his body would need at his ideal weight, he would have a calorie deficit of 240 calories a day or 1,680 calories a week, equaling a weight loss of about 1/2 pound a week. Once he reaches his ideal weight, if he continues to exercise actively, he could maintain a healthy weight and eat even more than he does now.

The exercise regimen needed to burn an extra 500 calories a day is difficult for most of us to sustain. It would be the equivalent of briskly jogging about 5 miles in 1 hour or cycling 11 miles in 50 minutes. Losing only 1/2 pound a week isn't gratifying to anyone shedding excess weight, so I recommend an increase in exercise *and* adherence to the permanent-weight-loss diet. This is the fastest way to lose weight. The weight-loss diet helps reduce your risk of heart disease and cancer because you cut out excess fats. Exercise increases your body conditioning, improves your health and vigor, and lowers your risk of heart disease, osteoporosis and possibly cancer.

To begin your program, set a caloric goal for yourself that is 200 calories a day *less* than you are currently consuming. For a person who is 20 pounds overweight, this is about the number of calories you would need once you reach your ideal weight. *Increase* your exercise so you are burning an extra 300 calories a day. This results in a deficit of 500 calories a day (3,500 calories a week), which equals about 1 pound of fat disappearing from your body each week.

If you eat 2,100 calories a day now, plan to eat 1,900 calories a day until you have reached your desired weight. If you can't manage to include 300 calories of exercise in your daily schedule, include 200 calories of exercise and reduce your food by 300 calories. The weight-loss result will be the same.

If you need to lose more than 20 pounds, lose weight in increments. As a severely overweight person, you may reach a plateau at your new reduced weight where the 500-calorie deficit is sufficient to maintain your lowered weight. When this occurs, you no longer lose weight. Let's look at another example of a 210-pound sedentary person whose ideal weight is 150 pounds.

210 x 12 = 2,520 calories to maintain present overweight

Reducing the food intake by 500 calories means following a 2,020 calorie diet. Once this overweight person reaches 168 pounds, he won't lose anymore weight because 2,020 calories is sufficient to maintain that weight.

168 x 12 = 2,020 calories

To reach 150 pounds, he will need to reduce his calories by another 500 calories. This is best achieved by eating 200 fewer calories and increasing exercise by 300 calories until the desired weight is reached.

If you are more than 20 pounds overweight, set your calorie and exercise goals for the first 20 pounds. You may not be physically fit enough to exercise vigorously if you are overweight. Be sure to consult your physician before beginning any diet or exercise program. Begin with significant calorie reduction, and add exercise gradually as you shed pounds, thus putting less strain on your heart.

Once you reach your first 20-pound goal, re-evaluate your caloric needs. Reduce them further and increase your exercise to begin on the next set of pounds. This gradual decrease in calorie consumption helps you adjust permanently to eating less, and you'll be able to maintain your weight loss once you reach your ideal weight.

If you wish to lose weight more rapidly than 1 pound a week, reduce your calories by even more than 300 fewer calories a day. But under no circumstances should you be eating less than 1,200 calories a day. Fewer calories than this cannot provide you with the nutrients your body needs every day. If you want to lose weight permanently, you increase your risk of breaking the diet if you do not eat wisely. You may feel hungry and deprived, angry and frustrated even as you see the pounds shed. Then you're more likely to break the diet, binge and gain back the weight you've lost. Take it slowly and steadily. Make gradual changes that become lifetime eating habits.

WHAT DO YOU EAT WHEN DIETING?

Your weight-loss diet should be a nutritionally sound program based on the principles of the risk-reducing nutrition plan. Eat foods high in complex carbohydrates and low in protein and fat, with plenty of fiber. Incorporate into your weight-loss program the proportions of 65% carbohydrates, 20% fat and 15% protein that define the risk-reducing nutrition plan. You'll be cutting down on unnecessary, fattening fats and proteins and emphasizing healthier, non-fattening carbohydrates.

By basing your weight-loss diet on the principles of the nutrition plan, you learn a nutritious way of eating you can follow for the rest of your life. You'll be making changes in your eating habits that become the core of maintaining your weight loss permanently.

On many fad diets, you eat some unappetizing foods and unusual food combinations that leave you feeling deprived. Once you've lost the pounds, you return to your former—and fattening—eating habits. Not with the permanent weight-loss diet!

With this diet, the foods you eat while dieting are the same foods you eat when you're transformed into the healthier, slimmer you. You learn a lifetime eating plan that helps you shed pounds and keep them off. The foods you eat are nourishing and good for your health—not a high-fat, high-protein diet that increases your risk of cancer and heart disease.

While losing weight and lowering your caloric intake, there's no room for empty calories. Avoid alcohol, and skip cake, candy, ice cream and soft drinks. Watch out for hidden fat and hidden calories. Stay away from fried foods, red meat and whole-milk dairy products. Go easy on margarine and salad dressings.

By doing this, you can easily lower your caloric intake by 200 calories a day. Those 200 calories are equal to about 1-1/2 tablespoons of butter, margarine or oil, or the fat in a 5-ounce hamburger, an 8-ounce sirloin steak or a 3-ounce piece of cheddar cheese. It's also equal to 1-1/2 soft drinks or 12 teaspoons of sugar.

To help during your weight-loss program, try the following ideas. Eat only at mealtimes. If it's not mealtime, stay out of the kitchen. Start the day with a substantial breakfast. Try to include high-fiber cereals and two fruits. Don't shortchange your body in the morning to save calories; a hearty breakfast satisfies you and reduces your need for eating later in the day.

Avoid business lunches because they often mean drinks—empty calories—and a full-course meal. Conduct your business in the office or while taking a walk—not in a restaurant. Your waistline and your health will appreciate it.

You must also change the eating habits that caused you to gain weight. To eat less, you must be aware of when you eat and why you eat. Try to understand the reasons you overate. Did the pounds slowly creep up from lack of physical activity? Are you using food as an emotional release? When the kids get you angry, do you open the pantry and have a bite? When you're bored, do you go to the refrigerator for a snack? Does eating relieve your anxiety? Do you eat when you're depressed?

Overeating—and getting fat—makes you more depressed and anxious; nothing gets resolved. During past diets, you probably did fine until a moment of crisis arose, causing you to break your diet and destroy your resolve. If you can recognize *now* what the emotional factors are that led you to overeat, you can head them off before they occur. Learn to handle these emotional issues that result in overeating, and you'll be less likely to break your diet.

WHY DO YOU WANT TO LOSE WEIGHT?

Short-term crash diets have a high-failure rate, and long-term, sensible diets are not easy to follow. Most overweight people try to lose weight—again and again. Many people start to diet because of external pressures—summer on the beach or jibes from friends or family. You try a quick-weight-loss diet, and the pressure of losing weight is alleviated. You please your spouse because you're dieting. The crash diet requires you to deprive yourself for several weeks, but you've lost the weight and everyone is happy—until you slowly begin to put it back on.

The effort to lose weight can be sustained for the short-term when the reason for losing outweighs the loss of the pleasures of eating. A young woman facing a walk down the aisle will manage to lose weight to fit into the wedding gown of her choice and size. A young boxer is able to get down to a certain weight to qualify for a fight. But should the wedding plans sour or the boxer get the 10 count, both dieters will regain the weight they lost. Their inability to reach their goal will be the excuse needed to return to undesirable eating habits.

Or if they do reach their goals, the bride and the boxer may soon resume old eating habits. Food may be considered a reward for reaching the intended goal!

Don't let this happen to you. Your goal must be merely to look better to please yourself and to protect your health. Only then will you have the willpower to stick to it and change lifelong bad eating habits into lifelong good eating habits. If your goal is more than this—if you equate losing weight as a means to other successes—you are doomed to failure.

If you dislike the way you look or feel, think about that image each time you're about to eat. You have to want to change that appearance or feeling to be successful.

Halfhearted dieting won't work. You need to be determined—that's willpower!

Many people believe they have no willpower to stay on a diet, and they set themselves up for failure. In reality, your lack of willpower is based on an image of yourself as weak and self-indulgent when it comes to dealing with food. If you begin a diet assuming the worst, it's natural for you to follow through and act the way you anticipate. This attitude protects you from having to change because you believe you're weak and can't help it.

You *aren't* weak unless you make yourself that way by setting unrealistic goals to be achieved by fraudulent methods. Bolster your self-image through therapy, if necessary. Decide to change now; you can do it if you want to.

CHANGE YOUR HABITS

You *can* change your eating habits. Don't get discouraged if you find it difficult because it will be. Take your time; this is a long-term project. Approach it slowly because you are no longer looking for a weight loss of 5 pounds in a week. Perhaps for a while you shouldn't get on the scale. Forget about losing weight; instead concentrate on changing your eating patterns.

Begin controlling your food intake at the supermarket. Don't buy what you shouldn't eat; that's the easiest way to avoid temptation. When you buy groceries, make sure you purchase only what you should be eating. If you can't avoid temptation at the grocery store, let someone else do the shopping.

Skip foods you can avoid. Say no to a cocktail or cheese and crackers before dinner. Have a salad instead of a hot lunch. If you can't bring yourself to go for the salad right away, at least skip the gravy. Bit by bit, wean yourself from your long-established habits. Try to avoid business lunches and dinners. Ease yourself out of your old patterns.

Within a few weeks or a few months, you'll find you have less desire for the foods you once ate. Your focus on food will diminish as you center your lifestyle on other activities and pursuits.

It's a good idea to establish a schedule of eating at specific times. The less often you eat, the better. Two and a half meals is best for most people. Try a full breakfast, a small lunch and a light dinner.

Each time you put food in your stomach, your digestive system starts working. The more your digestive system is stimulated, the more it transmits hunger signals to the brain. That's why snacking may increase your appetite. Frequent, small feedings work in laboratory animals where the food offered is controlled, but for humans with access to hamburgers, soda, ice cream and candy bars, frequent snacks are counter-productive. The less you tempt yourself, the better.

We think about food too much and too often. Once you start the digestive process, you become hungry, and feeling hungry, you eat. The cycle develops, and you become an obsessive overeater. The effect is emotional and physical. To break the addiction, you must constantly re-examine your eating habits.

Make eating less of a reflex action. Dieting and deciding what to eat must be a conscious effort. Satisfy your hunger within realistic limits of good nutrition and low caloric intake. Pay attention to what you eat. Don't get caught up in a conversation and take a second helping by accident.

Eating in a restaurant may be difficult. It's harder to select foods that are good for you, but you can do it. Ask the waiter to take the butter off the table. Order a smaller portion of meat, and ask for a larger serving of vegetables. Be assertive. Create a new lifestyle for yourself.

If you must eat out and have difficulty controlling your diet, compensate for it at home. If you've gone off your diet for one meal, don't use this as an excuse to go back to old habits. If you ate more than you should have, make up for it by eating less at the next meal or two. Try to eat as many meals at home as possible; it's easier to control your food intake.

Most overweight people are psychologically normal. The answer lies in learning to break bad eating habits and junk-food addictions. You can do this if you really want to. The answer to the question, "To diet or not to diet?" is up to you. If you want to lose weight to improve your health and appearance for your own sake, you can do it.

MAINTAIN YOUR WEIGHT LOSS

Once you reach your desired weight, don't feel you can binge or stop exercising. It's doubtful you will because you won't have felt terribly deprived of food during your diet, and the exercise will be a part of your life now. Once you reach your ideal weight, calculate how many calories you need to sustain your weight at the exercise level you choose, and don't exceed it. This may mean you can eat as many calories as you were before dieting *as long as you exercise.*

To be sure pounds don't slowly creep back on, weigh yourself every morning. If you find you've gained a few pounds, watch your calories for the next few weeks. Don't drink any wine, beer or liquor. Say no to desserts and pastries, and try to avoid restaurants.

With my permanent-weight-loss diet, you won't dramatically shed pounds and inches, but after several months you'll look and feel better. By slowly altering your eating and exercise habits, you'll make permanent changes in your lifestyle that result in permanent weight loss. These changes are good for your health and well-being, as well as for your figure.

You are learning a new, healthier way of eating and exercising, and you're letting go of your old ways. Keep working at your new lifestyle program. With diligent effort, thought and planning, you can lose weight and keep it off without endangering your health.

17.

HOW EXERCISE REDUCES YOUR RISK

*TAKE THIS TEST TO MEASURE YOUR
ACTIVITY LEVEL*

This test measures how active you are in your daily life. Circle the score for each characteristic that applies to you. Calculate the score, as shown on page 217, then check your activity category on page 218.

1. During your job or occupation you:
    1. Sit or stand, rarely walk
    2. Sit or stand most of the time, but get up and walk around once an hour
    3. Walk around most of the day
    4. Walk around and perform vigorous activity

2. You get to your job by:
    1. Private or public vehicle with minimal walking
    2. Private or public vehicle with several blocks of walking
    3. Walking or biking 1/4 to 1/2 mile
    4. Walking or biking more than 1/2 mile

3. How many times do you walk up a flight of stairs each day?
    1. None
    2. 1 to 3 times

3. 4 to 6 times
4. 7 or more times

4. You do housework, such as sweeping, vacuuming and scrubbing:
   1. Less than once a week
   2. Once a week
   3. 2 times a week
   4. 3 times a week or more

5. When you do housework, you usually work:
   1. Slowly and methodically, cleaning one room at a time
   2. Slowly and methodically, cleaning the whole house
   3. Rapidly, cleaning one room at a time
   4. Rapidly, cleaning the entire house

6. When you do laundry, you usually:
   1. Put all the clothes in the dryer
   2. Put some of the clothes in the dryer and hang some up to dry
   3. Hang most of the clothes up and put some in the dryer
   4. Hang all the clothes up to dry

7. You do heavy yard work, such as mowing, raking, digging or shoveling snow:
   1. Less than once a week
   2. Once a week
   3. 2 times a week
   4. 3 times a week or more

8. When you drive someplace, such as to a shopping center, you usually:
   1. Drive around or wait until there is a parking space close to the entrance
   2. Park as close as possible without waiting
   3. Take the first parking space you see
   4. Park at the end of the lot to give yourself a little walk

9. When you shop for groceries you:
   1. Drive directly to the store and methodically go up and down each aisle selecting your purchases
   2. Drive directly to the store, go up and down the aisles and often backtrack to make all your selections
   3. Walk several blocks to a store
   4. Walk several blocks and go from store to store to make all your purchases.

10. When you have a nearby errand to do you:
    1. Drive there
    2. Usually drive but sometimes walk there

3. Occasionally drive but usually walk there
4. Always walk there

11. During the evenings or non-working hours you usually:
    1. Watch television or read
    2. Go shopping or work on a craft or hobby
    3. Do house or yard work
    4. Go for a walk

12. When you walk at your job and when shopping, you usually walk:
    1. Slowly, at an unhurried pace
    2. At a moderate pace
    3. Briskly
    4. Briskly and sometimes even run

13. When you need something that's in another room, you usually:
    1. Ask someone to bring it to you
    2. Decide you can wait until later
    3. Wait until you have another reason to get up before getting it
    4. Go get it as soon as you realize you need the item

Calculating Your Score

Total the number of 1s, 2s, 3s and 4s. Then fill them in below, and do the indicated calculations. Add the scores together to determine your Total Score. Check your risk category on the following page.

_____ (1s) x 1 = _____

_____ (2s) x 2 = _____

_____ (3s) x 3 = _____

_____ (4s) x 4 = _____

Total Score _____

INTERPRETING YOUR SCORE

To determine your score, add all scores. Check your total score to see if your health and your life are at risk. You may be referred to the risk-reducing exercise plan, page 226.

13 to 19   **Extremely Sedentary**—You are extremely sedentary, which is putting your health at risk. Try to be more active. Begin the risk-reducing exercise plan now to lower your risk of heart disease, diabetes, cancer and osteoporosis.

20 to 30   **Sedentary**—You are too sedentary for good health. Try to be more active. Follow the risk-reducing exercise plan to lower your risk of heart disease, diabetes, cancer and osteoporosis.

31 to 45   **Moderately Active**—You are moderately active, and this gives you some protection. To help lower your risk of heart disease, cancer, diabetes and osteoporosis, follow the risk-reducing exercise plan.

46+   **Active**—Your daily activities provide an excellent amount of physical activity, but unless your occupation entails vigorous aerobic activity, follow the risk-reducing exercise plan. It offers you the maximum protection from heart disease, diabetes and cancer.

How Exercise Reduces Your Risk

People who are physically fit and engage in regular exercise throughout their lives have dramatically lower risks of heart disease, high blood pressure, sudden death and diabetes. Exercise also plays a role in protecting you from cancer! If you're physically active, you have a greater chance of surviving a heart attack than a sedentary person, and you're less likely to succumb to ill health earlier in life.

Throughout history, human beings have been physically active creatures. We have worked strenuously to maintain even a precarious existence. Only in recent history has the lifestyle of the majority of people in the Western world become sedentary. With a sedentary lifestyle has come increased rates of heart disease. The Industrial Revolution enabled us to move less and accomplish more, but it also meant we were no longer using our cardiovascular systems the way they were designed to be used.

The housewife or overworked executive who gets hooked on Valium or Librium might cope better if the doctor advised a long walk when stress becomes too much to bear. A brisk 15-minute walk does more to reduce muscle tension than a tranquilizer! Exercise burns up stress hormones and leaves you feeling relaxed.

EXERCISE DOES HAVE BENEFITS

The benefits of exercise accrue throughout your life. If you have always been physically active, you're better off than if exercise became a habit in later years. Exercising at any time in your life brings immediate benefits—as long as you keep at it. You can't simply sit back and "rest on the laurels" of previous commendable efforts. Exercise must be continued throughout your life or the benefits will dissipate rapidly.

Unlike money in the bank, where a deposit compounds interest automatically, you must keep investing exercise time to maintain the benefits of exercise. Fitness at 20 or 30 does not ensure fitness later in life; you have to keep at it.

Professional football players who run regularly and do hard workouts daily lose up to 50% of their conditioning with a 2- or 3-week layoff. But they quickly recoup their conditioning loss when they resume exercising. The older you are, the more quickly you lose physical fitness and the longer it takes to regain it. So it's best for those who wish to live longer and be healthier to exercise as regularly as possible.

Over a lifetime, a body that is exercised regularly will maintain itself in its youngest, healthiest state for the longest period of time. By exercising, you can achieve the sense of well-being necessary to be vigorous and energetic, and to develop confidence and poise. I can't promise you that leading a physically active life will confer immunity to ill health, but if you exercise regularly, you may significantly lower your risks of a range of ailments, such as hypertension, coronary disease, peptic ulcer, erratic diabetic control, low-back pain, stress, osteoporosis and cancer.

Beginning on page 226, I describe the risk-reducing exercise plan, which you can incorporate easily into your daily routine. Proper exercise and nutrition are the two keys to the risk-reducing program described in this book.

But first, I want to present you with the research facts behind this program because carefully analyzed studies of thousands of people demonstrate those who are physically active throughout their lives have better chances of avoiding ill health. Furthermore, if you're an active person and develop an illness, you have a better chance of surviving and recovering.

Though doctors and researchers have suspected for years that exercise is an important factor in preventing heart disease and perhaps cancer, conclusive evidence has only recently been demonstrated. Dr. Ralph Paffenberger, an internationally famous epidemiologist working at Stanford University Medical Center, recently published the results of an important study. He followed 17,000 Harvard alumni, ages 35 to 84, for up to 10 years. He evaluated their exercise habits, among other lifestyle choices, in relation to heart disease, sudden death and other illnesses. He found there were significantly fewer deaths from all causes, including cancer and cardiovascular disease, among men who exercised regularly. When the most sedentary men were matched with those who exercised the most, there was a 200% increase in death from cardiovascular disease.

The Harvard study that Paffenberger was involved in also showed that patients who were active after a heart attack were 33% less likely to suffer a second attack than those who are inactive. Men who were inactive during the college years who took up exercise later in life had a significantly lower risk when compared to college athletes who became sedentary.

Paffenberger concluded that if an individual increased his physical activity to a high level, he would lower his risk of coronary disease by 25%. If he stopped smoking, the risk was lowered by 25%. If high blood pressure was lowered, the risk was reduced by 16%. By increasing exercise and stopping smoking, the risk of heart disease was lowered by 30%.

The critical amount of exercise seemed to be an expenditure of at least 2,000 calories of exercise a week. The best risk-reduction was achieved by an expenditure of over 3,000 calories of exercise a week, with bursts of vigorous activity in the exercise. These men achieved a 50% reduction in risk from heart-disease-related deaths.

Similar results were demonstrated in another study by Dr. Paffenberger in which he followed 12,000 San Francisco longshoremen for over 20 years. This study compared vigorously active, moderately active and inactive men between the ages of 35 and 84. The conclusions demonstrate a convincing *doubled risk* of heart attack and a *tripled risk* of sudden death from heart attack among those in the low-activity category compared to those in the high-activity category.

Other studies also point to the protective effects of exercise Research in New York

City by Dr. E. Frank followed 55,000 men aged 25 to 64. Data showed when heart attacks did occur, sedentary victims were 3 times more likely to die than physically active victims.

A study by the London School of Hygiene and Tropical Medicine, conducted by Professor J. Morris, followed 18,000 civil-service workers for 8 years. It showed vigorous exercise performed only on weekends gave a benefit of 50% fewer heart problems than no vigorous exercise at all. The protection was demonstrable for men of all ages, even those in their 70s, despite the presence of other coronary risk factors.

A study of life expectancy conducted by Drs. Breslow and Belloc on nearly 7,000 adults in Alameda, California, compared patterns of unhealthy habits to healthy habits, such as regular exercise, not smoking, moderate alcohol consumption, reasonable weight, good eating habits and regular, sound sleep. This study demonstrated that healthy habits do increase longevity; results depended on age and how closely good habits were followed. For example, a 45-year-old man who observed all the above health practices could expect to live another 33 years, to the age of 78, while a similar man who only observed two or three of the healthy living habits could expect to live only 21 more years, to the age of 66.

Just statistics, right? Yes, but you only pass this way once, so why not have the odds in your favor? These research results should be enough to convince you to get out of your easy chair and engage in some exercise.

CAN EXERCISE BE RISKY?

We've all heard stories of a high-school track star who dropped dead after a meet. Or the story of a man who died on the golf course whose doctor, just the day before, had declared him physically fit. Jim Fixx, the well-known runner and author of *The Complete Book of Running,* died of a massive heart attack. These tragedies happen, and we hear about them because the media sensationalizes such ironic events. But if you choose to use such incidents as an excuse for not exercising, you're making the wrong choice. It won't happen to you if you get a thorough checkup that includes the proper medical tests *before* you begin an exercise program.

Studies of sudden death show that in men over age 30, 90% of the deaths were due to coronary disease, which is usually diagnosable. In those under 30, 80% of the deaths were caused by a congenital structural defect called *hypertrophic-cardiomyopathy,* which is also diagnosable, though often not suspected or looked for in ordinary physical examinations.

A young person contemplating vigorous sports should have a complete cardiologic exam to rule out any such unlikely, but tragic, problems.

The incidences described above are unusual and probably preventable. The track star may have suffered from a rare congenital heart defect. There are a range of "silent" conditions that may go undiagnosed because they are symptomless until a fatal or near-fatal situation puts extra stress on the heart. A defect within the mitral or aortic valve of the heart can result in sudden death in an apparently healthy high-school track star. Even a sudden energetic golf swing can produce a tear of a vulnerable heart valve cord and result in critical heart failure.

Jim Fixx had major risk factors of heart disease, despite his exercise habits. He had once been a heavy smoker. He ate a high-cholesterol, high-fat diet. His father died at 43 of a second heart attack. Fixx apparently ignored the many warning signs that forewarned of the attack, and he refused to undergo a stress test, which would have identified his risks.

I have observed this attitude myself in marathon runners, and it has been confirmed in studies done by Dr. E. Colt of St. Lukes Hospital in New York City. He notes among victims of sudden cardiac arrest "a reluctance to stop running despite warning symptoms." These runners ignored or denied their discomfort until they succumbed to a heart attack.

TAKE A STRESS TEST

Whatever you've been doing without difficulty up to now you can probably continue to do without risk. But the older you get, and the greater the number of risk factors you have, the greater the chance you may develop some degree of unsuspected coronary-artery disease. Only 1% of all people under age 35 have heart problems, but even the healthy heart has limitations on its capacity to pump blood and increase its rate of beating.

To protect yourself from exercise-related tragedies due to hidden heart disease, it's a good idea to have a complete physical exam, along with special tests, *before* you begin an increased exercise program. Have your heart checked for conditions known to cause collapse, such as rhythm disorders, structural valve and muscle abnormalities and clogged coronary arteries.

The amount of stress that can be placed on your heart and cardiovascular system varies with your age, physical condition and genetics. Generally the younger, trimmer and more active you are, the greater your heart's ability to tolerate stress. If you've been active all your life, it's probably safe to keep up the same level of activity as you grow older.

If you're planning to increase your exercise or take up vigorous running or other strenuous activities, have a maximum stress test, especially if you're over 35. This test observes the effects of strenuous effort on your heart. Excessive strain can cause changes in your heart's electrical rhythms, compromising its function. This can only be observed during a stress test performed while you're exercising—there's no other way of diagnosing it. Even someone with a heart condition may have a normal EKG reading when lying quietly on a doctor's examination table. "Silent" conditions may never be diagnosed unless studied under exertional stress.

Heart and cardiovascular disorders often develop slowly, without warning symptoms. It's advisable for anyone exercising regularly to have an annual stress test after age 40, especially if there's a history of high blood pressure, irregular heartbeats, chest discomfort or a family history of heart disease.

Examination during the rapid heart action that occurs with an exercise stress test is valuable in verifying your heart's stability. The effects of elevated blood pressure and rhythm disorders, as well as heart sounds, murmurs and clicks, can be observed. A stress test also determines the safe level at which you, at your age and fitness level, can start to exercise. This can help you avoid overexertion that could lead to collapse and possible death.

Along with a careful physical examination and a chest X-ray, stress testing can help evaluate whether exercising poses a risk to your heart. If it does, ambulatory monitoring (a 24-hour, continuous EKG recording) and echo cardiography (ultrasound picture of intracardiac structures) can further identify your potential risk.

Nearly everyone should be moving his muscles regularly, no matter what his state of health. Someone with high blood pressure or a precarious heart condition should not exert himself as much as a healthy person should. If you have health problems, consult your physician about your exercise capabilities and limitations. It's impossible to state categorically you can avoid sudden death or heart attack while exercising, regardless of your health. But odds are undeniably improved in your favor if you exercise wisely and regularly. Exercise builds healthy hearts and healthy bodies. You can feel confident about lowering your risk of ill health by engaging in a vigorous exercise program after clearance from your physician.

WHAT KIND OF EXERCISE REDUCES RISK?

There are three basic kinds of exercise—*isotonic, isometric* and *aerobic*—though many activities combine them.

Isotonic exercise, such as weight-lifting, tenses the muscles against a resistant or heavy force and tends to build muscle strength without improving your heart and cardiovascular system. *Isometric* exercise pits one muscle or part of the body against another or against an immovable object in a strong but motionless action, such as pressing, pushing or pulling.

The extreme tension in the muscles caused by isotonic and isometric exercises can have harmful effects. Blood vessels become constricted, impairing blood circulation and limiting the oxygen supply to the muscles being exercised. These exercises can put a pressure load on the heart muscle, injuring its structure and function, and can raise blood pressure alarmingly. Intense straining can harm even a healthy heart, and moderate straining can threaten a heart with a silent condition.

Aerobic exercise increases the body's demand for oxygen because large groups of muscles are used and demand more oxygen. The heart must beat faster to furnish this

223

extra oxygen; in this situation, the heart's muscle tone and pumping action are improved.

With regular aerobic exercise, the muscles and organs use oxygen more efficiently, and the heart develops a stronger beat with increased blood pumped in every stroke. It beats less frequently to supply the needed blood and oxygen, so your pulse rate is lowered. The objective benefits of aerobic exercise can be measured by increased endurance.

The end result of regular aerobic exercise is a better functioning body and better psyche. Your heart pumps more efficiently and uses less oxygen to perform the same amount of work. Your muscles extract oxygen from the blood more easily. Your intestines function more regularly, and you operate at a brighter psychological state with heightened creativity and an increased feeling of well-being.

In an aerobically conditioned body, stress hormones (catecholamines), which your body produces in response to tension, fear, anger or anxiety, are more easily dissipated. This results in less heart stimulation and a reduced feeling of tension. You experience fewer stress symptoms, such as palpitations, tension headaches, muscle aches, high blood pressure, diarrhea, gas or constipation.

Aerobic exercise also protects your heart by increasing the blood levels of "protective" HDL cholesterol in relation to the undesirable LDL cholesterol. A higher level of HDL cholesterol is associated with a lower risk of coronary atherosclerosis and heart attack.

An important study of how exercise affects coronary atherosclerosis was recently published in the *New England Journal of Medicine*. Researchers used monkeys bred to develop coronary atherosclerosis when they were fed a high-fat diet. One group was kept sedentary; the other group was given regular exercise. Results confirmed what we have long suspected in humans—the sedentary monkeys developed advanced coronary disease and experienced a high rate of sudden death. The monkeys in the exercised group were healthier, with fewer lesions in the heart and wider coronary arteries. They had a lower overall serum-cholesterol level and a higher HDL-cholesterol level.

Another benefit of aerobic exercise is improved control of serum-glucose levels. Exercise encourages increased uptake of glucose by the muscles, combined with an increased sensitivity to insulin, in normal and diabetic people. After 20 minutes of aerobic exercise, your body switches from burning primarily carbohydrates for energy to burning more fat. If you are a trained athlete—or in top condition from regular vigorous exercise—your body adapts by using fat for energy and storing the carbohydrates in the muscles and liver for use in endurance activities.

The combination of a sensible exercise-and-nutrition program may control hypoglycemia and some forms of hyperglycemia by keeping blood-sugar levels within the normal range, resulting in better control of weight and emotions. The person with high blood sugar (hyperglycemia), due to dietary overconsumption or defective handling of blood glucose, benefits from a regular exercise program because exercise helps normalize the blood-sugar levels by increasing its utilization.

The most beneficial forms of aerobic exercise are those in which the arms and legs are in constant motion with minimal resistance, such as running, cross-country skiing, swimming, cycling and dancing. Other sports, including basketball, football and tennis, offer varying degrees of aerobic exercise, but the amount of aerobic activity is less than the activities mentioned above. The benefits of football, for example, depend on the position played. A wide receiver who frequently sprints downfield receives more aerobic exercise than the center or place kicker. A tennis match may provide little or no aerobic activity if points are scored quickly as a result of well-placed serves.

Some sports and exercise activities combine aerobic and muscle-strengthening exercise. Although this is desirable from the standpoint of improving physical attractiveness, the muscle-strengthening aspect is less important. The ultimate goal of exercising is to increase the level of cardiovascular fitness and to maintain it. This need not be achieved through obsessive long-distance running. The amount of exercise you need to include in your weekly routine to achieve cardiac fitness is probably less than you think. It doesn't have to be exceedingly time-consuming; hopefully it will be fun and rewarding. You don't need to engage in competitive sports unless you want to. Anything that increases your body's motion and increases your heart rate will work.

By exercising regularly, you can slow the deterioration that comes with aging. You can help improve circulation to your vital organs, help lower artery-clogging serum-cholesterol levels and help open the tiny capillaries that feed your muscles, brain, heart, lungs, spinal cord, nerves and other organs. An optimally functioning cardiovascular system supplies more blood to your brain, kidneys, heart, spinal cord, digestive system, sexual organs and muscles, and they function at their highest level. You'll feel better, look better and have more energy when you exercise regularly. Most important, exercise reduces your risk of diseases that strike many down in their prime.

18.

THE RISK-REDUCING EXERCISE PLAN

*TAKE THIS TEST TO MEASURE YOUR
EXERCISE PROGRAM*

This test evaluates the exercise program in which you regularly participate. Circle the score for each characteristic that applies to you. Calculate the score, then check your risk category on pages 227 and 228.

Frequency of Exercise

Choose one.
You allocate time for exercise:
+ 5   Daily or almost daily
+ 4   3 to 5 times a week
+ 3   2 times a week
+ 2   Once a week
+ 1   Less than 3 times a month

Intensity of Exercise

Choose one.

The kind of exercise you do requires:

+5   Sustained, vigorous activity
+4   Intermittent, vigorous activity
+3   Sustained, moderately vigorous activity
+2   Intermittent, moderately vigorous activity
+1   Light, leisurely activity

Duration of Exercise

Choose one.

Your exercise routine lasts approximately:

+4   45 minutes or longer
+3   20 to 40 minutes
+2   10 to 20 minutes
+1   less than 10 minutes

Calculating Your Score

Multiply the three scores together:

$$\underline{\hspace{2cm}} \text{ X } \underline{\hspace{2cm}} \text{ X } \underline{\hspace{2cm}} = \underline{\hspace{2cm}}$$

Frequency   Duration   Intensity   Total Score

INTERPRETING YOUR SCORE

Check your total score below to see if your health and your life are at risk. You may be referred to the risk-reducing nutrition plan, page 186, or the risk-reducing exercise plan.

81 to 100   **Lowest Risk**—Your present activity level is optimum for reducing risk; coupled with the risk-reducing nutrition plan, it puts you at the lowest risk of developing a life-threatening illness.

61 to 80   **Low Risk**—Your present activity level is a healthy one, but it isn't as vigorous as it could be. Follow the risk-reducing nutrition plan, and continue your exercise routine to bring you the greatest benefits.

41 to 60   **Moderately Low Risk**—Your present level of activity offers you protective benefits, but increase the level of your exercise to provide greater protection. Follow the risk-reducing nutrition plan to assure maximum health.

31 to 40   **Moderate Risk**—You aren't getting enough exercise; this may be putting you at moderate risk of heart disease, stroke, diabetes and cancer, depending on other lifestyle choices. Follow the risk-reducing exercise plan and the risk-reducing nutrition plan to help lower your risks.

20 to 30   **High Risk**—Your exercise routine is inadequate for good health. You may be at high risk of developing heart disease, stroke, diabetes or cancer. Follow the risk-reducing exercise plan and the risk-reducing nutrition plan to help lower your risk.

Below 20   **Very High Risk**—Your exercise routine is totally inadequate for good health. You are probably at very high risk of developing heart disease, stroke, diabetes or cancer. Follow the risk-reducing exercise plan and the risk-reducing nutrition plan to help lower your risk.

The Risk-Reducing Exercise Plan

Based on medical evidence that clearly demonstrates the dramatic health benefits of exercise, I have devised a risk-reducing exercise plan to help lower your risk of heart attack, stroke, diabetes, osteoporosis and cancer. Follow this program *only after you have passed an exercise stress test and have been given the go-ahead by your physician.*

If you make exercise a part of your daily routine, it will soon become an enjoyable aspect of your life. You'll feel better physically and mentally, and you'll know you're taking positive measures to reduce your risk of disease.

The premise of this risk-reducing exercise plan is basic. The Harvard study found men who expended at least 2,000 calories a week in exercise showed they significantly benefited their cardiovascular systems. Those who expended 3,000 calories showed the greatest reduction of risks. Men who also included vigorous aerobic activities exhibited the greatest reduction in heart attacks and other illnesses, including cancer. You can reduce risks if you exercise enough to burn between 2,000 and 3,000 calories every week.

Even if you're a very busy person juggling job and family, this won't be as hard as you think. My plan helps you find time to exercise and makes it a pleasurable aspect of your life.

If you do housework or gardening and a normal amount of walking during your day, you're already probably burning 1,000 calories a week in non-vigorous exercise. At least you're moving your body. Your goal should be to include enough exercise to burn another 2,000 calories. About half of those calories should be vigorously used ones.

If you're very sedentary, you may not be using those 1,000 calories, so you need to find ways to include moderate exercise in your daily routine. Climb a few flights of stairs instead of taking the elevator—the time it takes to walk up or down is probably equaled by the time it takes to wait for the elevator. Park the car at the far end of the parking lot, and walk a little farther. Use errands as a stimulus to fitness rather than regarding them as an annoyance. There's no excuse not to be active!

If you have physical limitations, whether from a handicap or disease, try to include exercise in your weekly activities. Your doctor can advise you on suitable exercises. Even limited exercise has its benefits. Long, slow walks are useful for maintaining fitness for a cardiac or elderly person. But without vigorous exercise, fitness in a younger, healthy individual won't improve.

THE RISK-REDUCING EXERCISE PLAN

I want you to exercise *every day,* alternating between days of vigorous and non-vigorous activities. By exercising vigorously every other day, your muscles have time to recover from the previous day's strain and to store glycogen, which supplies energy to your muscles. This will also prevent you from getting "hooked" on exercise; some people use exercise as a panacea for whatever ails them.

For non-vigorous exercise—walk! Unless it's pouring rain, a blowing blizzard, over 95F (35C) or below 20F (-7C), you should walk. Dress wisely and appropriately for the weather, and you'll enjoy the change of seasons. If the weather is bad, find someplace indoors to walk. Covered shopping malls are good for extremely hot or cold weather, or try a sports arena at a local college or university. If you use your imagination, you'll be able to find a place to walk.

Easy walking (2mph) burns 210 calories an hour; brisk walking (3-3/4mph) burns 300 calories an hour. If you walk briskly for 1 hour a day, 4 days a week, including 5-minute warm-up and cool-down periods, you'll burn a total of 1,040 calories.

Walking helps release tension, and it can be a good activity in other ways. Make it a special time for you and your spouse—you'll both benefit from the exercise and the chance to talk with each other. Or walk with your children. Take one child at a time to give you the opportunity for sharing.

After burning 1,040 calories in 4 days of walking, you have 960 calories to expend in vigorous activities on the other 3 days. You can burn these calories with more aerobic-type activities, such as bicyling, swimming or jogging briskly. The chart below gives the approximate time you'll need to spend at each kind of exercise to burn 300 calories.

For vigorous exercise, choose an activity you enjoy, and it'll be easier to stay with it. If you're a social person, join an aerobics class or a fitness class. Swimming may be

Amount of Exercise Needed to Burn 300 Calories	
Housework	1 hour 35 minutes
Bicycling (5-1/2mph)	1 hour 25 minutes
Walking (2-1/2mph)	1 hour 25 minutes
Canoeing (2-1/2mph)	1 hour 15 minutes
Golf	1 hour 10 minutes
Mowing lawn (power mower)	1 hour 10 minutes
Walking (3-3/4mph)	1 hour
Rowing (2-1/2mph)	1 hour
Swimming (1/4mph)	1 hour
Volleyball	55 minutes
Square dancing	50 minutes
Tennis	45 minutes
Gardening (heavy digging)	45 minutes
Hiking uphill	35 minutes
Cross-country skiing (10mph)	30 minutes
Cycling (13mph)	30 minutes
Brisk jogging	30 minutes
Running (10mph)	15 minutes

Data is based on calories burned by a 150-pound person. If you weigh less, you'll burn fewer calories; if you weigh more, you'll burn more calories.

the best exercise—it is non-traumatic to joints. Racquetball or singles tennis can be good exercise, especially if you like a little competition to make the game interesting.

When suggesting exercise activities to my patients, I take into account their age, present fitness and health, and the type of exercise they like to do and can fit into their daily life. Exercise should be enjoyable. Your choices might include running, swimming, cycling, tennis, squash, badminton, volleyball, hiking, playing frisbee, cross-country skiing, touch football, basketball, soccer, hockey, field hockey, rowing, dancing or any other activity that increases motion and locomotion. Awareness of your physical condition is essential in determining the amount and type of exercise you should attempt.

If your reason for not exercising is that you're too busy, take another look! This is just an excuse. If driving to a fitness club takes too much time, exercise at home. An exercycle or rowing machine in your home is convenient, rain or shine, 24 hours a day, 365 days a year. It won't accept any excuses such as, "It's too cold today," or "I can't find a tennis partner."

If you can't "find" time, make it! Steal it from other activities. Row while watching the evening news or your favorite television show. Pedal the exercycle while you read or talk on the telephone. Get up 1/2 hour earlier to exercise, or shut the door to your spouse and family and say, "The next 30 minutes are mine!"

Don't rely on one kind of activity for your vigorous exercise. Variety is enjoyable, and it gives you alternatives if your racquetball partner has to work late, you develop shin splints or your exercise class is cancelled for the holidays.

Some people get hooked on exercise, particularly running. Research by Dr. Connie Chan, a psychologist at the University of Massachusetts, revealed joggers who had to stop jogging to recuperate from a sports injury became markedly depressed. Jogging had become their only mechanism for coping with stress. Without it, they were lost. No other exercise they performed, such as swimming or bicycling, improved their depression. Don't let this happen to you!

Exercise is your main objective, even in competitive sports,. Don't approach a game with the attitude you must win; choose a partner with the same attitude as yours. Don't exercise or engage in sports as a way to vent anger or aggression—you may overdo it and exert yourself beyond your heart's capacity. Stress hormones, coupled with the demands of *vigorous* exercise, may cause arrhythmias and vascular collapse.

YOU CAN EXERCISE SAFELY

Whatever exercise you choose, do it in three phases: warm-up, stress period and cool-down. This even goes for walking! By warming up for 5 minutes *before* you exercise vigorously, you avoid muscle strain and stress on your heart. A 5-minute cool down also protects your heart.

Begin with a 5-minute *warm-up period*. Extend your lower back and the backs of your thighs and calves, while breathing deeply. Rotate your arms, run slowly in place, and begin your exercise gradually. For example, after stretching for 5 minutes, a runner should move from a fast walk to a jog to actual running. After exercising gradually for about 5 minutes, then you're ready for sprinting during the stress period.

The greatest benefit to your cardiovascular system really comes from the *sprint periods,* which are periods of exercise when the heart rate is raised to at least 70% of its maximum capacity. For your heart's safety, this period should vary from 1 to 4 minutes, depending on your level of conditioning. After working at that level, slow your exercise speed for 1 or 2 minutes before sprinting again so you don't overwork your heart.

To determine your heart's maximum rate, subtract your age from the number 220 You should strive for at least 70% of your maximum heart rate. The formula is:

220 − age = X

70% of X is your target heart rate

X is divided by 6 to determine your heart rate for 10 seconds (60/6 = 10)

Count your pulse rate for 10 seconds

An example for a person 35 years old working at 70% of his maximum heart rate, taking his heart rate for *10 seconds,* would be:

220 − 35 = 185

185 x .7 (70%) = 130

130 divided by 6 = 21

This person would strive for a heart rate of 21 beats for 10 seconds, after working vigorously, to indicate he was working at the point he wanted.

To take your pulse after a sprint period, hold two fingers against your carotid artery, which is in your neck just under the jaw. Count the beats for 10 seconds, and see how close you are to your target heart rate.

Maintain your target heart rate for limited periods—1 to 4 minutes—then slow down your exercise rate. This doesn't mean a perfectly healthy heart can't safely exercise at 70% for longer, but don't do it without being certain of its "perfect" health. See the chart on the opposite page for a list of ages and target heart rates.

The length of the sprint period varies with your ability and conditioning. Unless you are fully conditioned, don't extend this period if you are breathing heavily. If you're moderately active, 2 to 4 minutes of stress time is sufficient, then slow down until your breath and strength return. Sprint for another 2 to 4 minutes. Repeat this pattern 4 to 6 times, and build up your stamina so you are eventually able to sprint for a total of 20 to 30 minutes during the sprint period.

After your warm-up and sprint periods, end with a 5-minute *cool-down period.* This time is very important but often overlooked. The time immediately following vigorous exercise is a particularly vulnerable time for the heart's rhythm system. The two heart-stimulating hormones, epinephrine and norepinephrine, are at high levels. A sudden stop in the muscle action can bring on painful cramps, lightheadedness,

Age	Maximum age-predicted heart rate	70% of maximum heart rate	Heart rate for 10 seconds at 70% of maximum heart rate
20	200	140	23
25	195	137	22
30	190	133	22
35	185	130	21
40	180	126	21
45	175	123	20
50	170	119	20
55	165	116	19
60	160	112	19
65	155	109	18
70	150	105	18

dizziness, nausea and critical heart arrhythmia if the heart's blood supply is obstructed due to cardiovascular disease. Don't stop exercising abruptly; slow down for 5 minutes or more into gradually less-vigorous activity.

Vary the intensity and duration of your workout according to your age and fitness. Work up to the time and intensity needed to expend about 300 calories. This may take 3 to 6 months, but don't get discouraged. As you continue to exercise, your performance ability will increase, and you can speed up the exercise pace, sprinting more often.

To reach your long-term goal of reducing your health risks, avoid temporarily increasing it! Set long-term goals, and don't expect too much of yourself in the beginning. It takes time.

Some weekend tennis players or early-morning joggers push themselves to their limits every time they hit the court or jogging track. But it's doubtful they achieve any greater protection by this excess zeal than less-vigorous exercisers. Your body reaches a point at which, unless you are a dedicated athlete in training, your fitness level is adequate for well-being. Maintenance levels of exercise keep your body fit. That's why the risk-reducing exercise plan limits the amount of exercise you need to do.

You also need to take care of yourself after exercising; saunas and steambaths may feel good, but they can be dangerous. Don't take a sauna or steambath after vigorous activity; your heart must work extra hard to pump blood to your skin's surface to keep your body cool. This is particularly stressful after vigorous exercise, and it raises your blood pressure.

Perspiration induced by saunas and steambaths could also seriously dehydrate you after sweat-inducing vigorous exercise. (You may not see perspiration on your skin in a dry sauna because it evaporates immediately.) You can safely enjoy a sauna or steambath when you have cooled down and you are breathing easily. After you spend time in a sauna, be sure you drink enough water to rehydrate yourself.

Don't exercise if you have any illness, especially a respiratory virus. This type of illness makes your lungs less efficient, and exercising vigorously puts an added strain on your circulatory system. Let yourself recover fully before you resume exercising, then ease back into it because you may be out of condition. *Never* smoke immediately before exercising because the increased carbon monoxide in your blood robs your heart and muscles of necessary oxygen.

You need to dress properly for exercising. Wear lightweight, unrestricting clothes during warm weather or in heated indoor facilities. Cotton or cotton-blends feel most comfortable.

During cold weather, wear *layers* of warm clothing—a down vest on top is ideal. Protect your hands, feet, face and ears with wool or down clothing until your circulation has adapted to the temperature. In cold, windy weather, wear a mask or scarf over your mouth to protect your lungs from the cold because cold temperatures can precipitate lung spasm, respiratory distress, heart irregularities and even coronary spasm. Don't exercise outdoors if the temperature is below 20F (-7C) or it is very windy.

Very warm, humid weather also puts a strain on your circulatory system, increasing the chance of dehydration, cramps, heat stroke and heat prostration. If the temperature is over 90F (35C), or hot and humid, exercise indoors where it's cooler or in an air-conditioned facility. If you can't walk one day, don't be concerned. If the weather keeps you idle for several days, choose an indoor activity, such as dancing, jumping rope or running in place, to keep exercising.

WATCH FOR WARNING SIGNS

If you follow my advice, and that of your physician, hopefully you won't experience any real discomfort while exercising. Push yourself a little, but don't push yourself over the limit to benefit from exercise. If you experience any of the following warning signs during (or immediately after) exercise, stop and consult your doctor.

A burning pain in the chest, whether it's over your heart or not, is a signal to stop and seek medical attention. It may be only indigestion, but why take a chance? Marathon runners have been victims of heart attack while running because they simply didn't pay attention to warning signs.

Other warning signs include dizziness or lightheadedness, which may mean the brain is not getting enough blood because the heart or vascular reflexes are unable to keep up with the demands of exercise. If you become dizzy, lie down until you're breathing easily and your head feels normal. You may not have warmed up enough, or your exercise was too intense or too long for your conditioning. If dizziness is extreme, see a doctor, and have him check your heart and your blood-pressure reactions on a stress test. Then limit the intensity of exercise until you are in better condition.

If you experience an irregular heartbeat or pulse, such as skipping a beat, extra beats or more rapid beating than seems usual for the amount of exercise you have done, have it checked by your doctor. Though it may be insignificant, sometimes an irregular heartbeat can be a clue to a serious heart condition.

Less-serious symptoms, such as a "charley-horse," a "stitch" in the side, cramps or giddiness, may mean you have worked harder than your fitness level. Exert yourself a little less until your fitness improves.

WHAT TO EAT AND DRINK

Some people worry that their appetite will increase and they'll gain weight if they exercise—this won't happen. As you burn more calories, you can also eat more to maintain your present weight. But your appetite won't increase to the point that you'll gain weight. Often the feeling of well-being created by exercising counteracts feelings of hunger brought on by stress, boredom or depression.

Eat properly to nourish your body, but forget the notion that protein means muscle power. You don't need extra protein to keep your muscles in good condition. Until recently, athletes and trainers believed the best meal to eat before a big game was a high-protein meal consisting of a large steak and little starch or water. We now know differently.

Athletic energy does not come from protein; it comes from carbohydrates and fats. An inadequate water supply during exercise hastens exhaustion, fatigue and collapse. The best foods for athletes are complex carbohydrates. If you follow the risk-reducing nutrition plan, page 186, you'll be in top shape to get the most out of your exercise program.

Drink plenty of water. Your fluid needs increase dramatically when you exercise, and water is essential for all muscular activity. The more vigorous the exercise, the more you perspire. It's best to drink *water,* not juice or soft drinks, *before, during* and *after* exercising. Studies show no matter how much water you drink before you exercise, you probably won't drink as much as you lose. Overhydration is not usually a problem, but dehydration can be a very serious problem, especially if warm weather or excessive clothing contributes to water loss.

Commercial thirst quenchers offer no benefit to you. In fact, sugar-containing liquids may be the cause of cramps and diarrhea. Sugar may hasten exhaustion.

You get all the sodium, potassium and other salts you need from your diet, unless you perspire excessively during exercise. Your body is able to conserve potassium, and little is lost through perspiration.

Salt tablets, taken on the mistaken assumption you need to replace lost salts, are dangerous. The only time you need salt is when you've exceeded sensible exercise and you risk heat stroke. This may happen in rare cases, such as playing football in full uniform or running in rubber sweatsuits in hot, humid weather.

If you burn between 2,000 and 3,000 calories a week exercising, you're on the way to a healthier, more-fulfilling life. Coupled with a healthy diet, exercise makes you feel like a new person. It can help you feel better, look better and perform better.

APPENDIX

MISCELLANEOUS

	PORTION	FAT		PROTEIN		CARB.		KCAL
		grams	%	grams	%	grams	%	
Coleslaw	1c.	0.5	0.68	1.5	0.05	8.5	0.27	125
Cola	1c.	0	0	0	0	24	1	96
Fish sticks	1	3	0.49	5	0.36	2	0.15	55
Gelatin, sweetened	1c.	0	0	3.6	0.10	34	0.90	150
Ginger ale	1 oz.	0	0	0	0	18	1	72
Gingerbread	1 slice	4.3	0.22	2	0.04	32.2	0.74	174
Ice cream:								
regular	1c.	14	0.48	6	0.09	28	0.43	262
soft-serve	1c.	18	0.48	8	0.09	36	0.43	338
Potato chips	1 oz.	11	0.60	2	0.05	14	0.34	163
Pudding	1c.	1	0	2.50	0.10	20	0.81	99
Sherbet	1c.	2	0.07	2	0.03	59	0.90	262
Vanilla wafers	10	5	0.32	2	0.06	22	0.62	141
Wines	6 oz.	0	0	tr.	tr.	2	0.20	41

FATS & SUGARS

	PORTION	FAT		PROTEIN		CARB.		KCAL
		grams	%	grams	%	grams	%	
Avocado	1/4	9	0.82	1	0.04	3.5	0.14	99
Apple butter	1t.	tr.	tr.	tr.	tr.	8	0.97	33
Bacon, crisp	1 slice	4	0.69	3	0.23	1	0.08	52
Butter	1t.	6	0.98	tr.	tr.	tr.	tr.	55
Margarine	1t.	6	0.98	tr.	tr.	tr.	tr.	55
Cream, whipping								
40% Fat	1T.	6	0.97	tr.	tr.	tr.	tr.	56
20% Fat	1T.	5	0.96	tr.	tr.	tr.	tr.	47
Dressings:								
French	1T.	6	0.80	tr.	tr.	3	0.18	66
Italian	1T.	6	0.82	tr.	tr.	3	0.18	66
mayonnaise	1T.	12	0.98	tr.	tr.	tr.	tr.	110
mayonnaise-type	1T.	6	0.87	tr.	tr.	2	0.13	62
Roquefort	1T.	8	0.90	1	0.05	1	0.05	80
Dressings, low-calorie:								
French, Italian	1T.	2	0.82	tr.	tr.	1	0.18	22
Jam	1T.	tr.	tr.	tr.	tr.	14	0.98	57
Jelly	1T.	tr.	tr.	tr.	tr.	14	0.98	57
Peanuts	1T.	4	0.85	2	0.15	2	0.15	52
Pecans	1T.	5	0	1	0.07	1	0.08	53
Sugar	1T.	0	0.87	0	0	12	1	48
Walnuts	1T.	5	0.87	1	0.08	1	0.08	52
Oil	1T.	14	0.95	0	0	0	0	126
Olives	4	2	0	tr.	tr.	tr.	tr.	19
Vinegar	1T.	0	0	0	0	2	0.88	9

STARCHES & BREADS

	PORTION	FAT		PROTEIN		CARB.		KCAL
		grams	%	grams	%	grams	%	
Biscuits	1	6	0.38	3	08	17	0.48	140
Bread crumbs	1/2c.	2	0.10	5	0.12	32	0.77	166
Bread sticks, small	5	2	0.09	6	0.12	37	0.77	192
Bread, white	1 slice	1	0.13	2	0.12	12	0.73	65
Bread, whole-wheat	1 slice	1	0.14	2	0.13	11	0.72	61
Bun, hamburger	1 bun	2	0.15	3	0.10	21	0.73	114
Bun, hot-dog	1 bun	2	0.15	3	0.10	21	0.73	114
Cake, angel-food (small slice)	1	tr.	tr.	3	0.10	24	0.87	110
Cake, pound (small slice)	1	9	0.55	2	0.05	14	0.38	145
Cereal, dry unsweetened	1 oz.	tr.	tr.	2	0.07	24	0.87	110
Cereal cooked	1/2c.	1	0.12	3	0.17	12	0.68	70
Corn on cob	1 ear	1	0.10	3	0.14	16	0.75	85
Corn muffins	1	5	0.30	3	0.08	23	0.61	150
Cornstarch	1T.	tr.	tr.	tr.	tr.	7	0.93	30
Crackers								
graham, small sq.	4	1	0.16	1	0.07	10	0.72	55
oyster	10	1	0.21	1	0.09	7	0.68	41
round	5	4	0.41	2	0.09	10.5	0.48	86
rye	2	tr.	tr.	2	0.16	10	0.83	48
saltine	6	2	0.25	2	0.11	11	0.62	70
Flour, all-purpose	1T.	tr.	tr.	1	0.15	5.2	0.80	26
Pasta, cooked	1c.	1	0.04	6	0.12	39	0.82	189
Muffin	1	5	0.31	4	0.11	20	0.56	141
Noodles, egg, cooked	1c.	2	0.09	7	0.14	37	0.76	194
Pancake, wheat, 4''	1	2	0.29	2	0.12	9	0.58	62
Parsnips	1/2c.	0.50	0.07	1	0.07	11	0.77	57
Potato, baked	1	tr.	tr.	3	0.12	21	0.87	96
Potato, boiled	1	tr	tr.	2	0.10	18	0.90	80
Popcorn, unbuttered	1c.	3	0.41	1	0.06	8	0.49	65
Pretzel, small sticks	5	tr.	tr.	tr.	tr.	4	0.80	20
Pumpkin	1c.	1 00	0.10	2	0.08	18	0.80	89
Rice, grits	1c.	tr.	tr.	3	0.06	41	0.88	185
Roll, hard	1	2	0.11	5	0.12	31	0.76	162
Sesame seeds	1T.	2	0.72	1	0.16	0.5	0.08	25
Spaghetti, cooked	1c.	1	0.05	5	0.12	32	0.82	155
Squash, winter	1c.	1	0.05	4	0.10	32	0.83	153
Waffles	1	7	0.31	7	0.13	28	0.55	203
Wheat germ	4T.	2	0.22	4.5	0.22	8	0.39	81
Yams, baked, 6 oz.	1	1	0.05	2	0.05	36	0.92	155

MILK PRODUCTS

	PORTION	FAT		PROTEIN		CARB.		KCAL
		grams	%	grams	%	grams	%	
Buttermilk, skim	1c.	tr.	tr.	9	0.40	13	0.59	88
Milk:								
evaporated, skim	1/2c.	tr.	tr.	9	.42	12	0.57	84
evaporated, whole	1/2c.	10	0.51	9	0.20	12	0.27	174
non-fat dry, mixed	1c.	tr.	tr.	9	0.40	13	0.59	88
non-fat dry, powder	1/2c.	tr.	tr.	12	0.40	18	0.59	122
skim	1c.	tr.	tr.	9	0.40	13	0.59	88
butterfat 1%	1c.	3	0.26	8	0.31	12	0.47	101
butterfat 2%	1c.	5	0.37	8	0.26	12	0.39	121
whole	1c.	12	0.60	9	0.20	9	0.20	180
Yogurt, 2% butterfat	1c.	4	0.30	8	0.26	13	0.43	120

VEGETABLES

	PORTION	FAT		PROTEIN		CARB.		KCAL
		grams	%	grams	%	grams	%	
Asparagus	1/2c.	tr.	tr.	2	0.40	3	0.60	20
Green beans	1/2c.	tr.	tr.	1	0.25	3	0.75	16
Bean sprouts	1/2c.	1	0.31	3	0.41	2	0.27	29
Beets	1/2c.	tr.	tr.	1	0.14	6	0.85	28
Broccoli	1/2c.	tr.	tr.	2.5	0.40	4	0.64	26
Brussels sprouts	1/2c.	0.50	0.14	2.5	0.32	4	0.51	31
Cabbage	1/2c.	tr.	tr.	0.5	0.25	1.5	0.75	8
Carrots, raw	1/2c.	tr.	tr.	0.5	0.07	6.5	0.92	28
Cauliflower	1/2c.	tr.	tr.	1.5	0.33	3	0.66	18
Celery	1/2c.	tr.	tr.	0.5	0.20	2	0.80	10
Chicory	1/2c.	tr.	tr.	1	0.16	3	0.48	25
Cucumber	1/2c.	tr.	tr.	0.5	0.12	3.5	0.87	16
Eggplant	1/2c.	tr.	tr.	1	0.20	4	0.80	20
Endive	1/4c.	tr.	tr.	1	0.33	2	0.66	12
Escarole	1/4c.	tr.	tr.	1	0.33	2	0.66	12
Greens, mixed	1/2c.	0.50	0.08	2	0.26	5	0.66	30
Lettuce, iceberg	1/3 head	tr.	tr.	1	0.20	4	0.80	20
Mushrooms, canned	1/2c.	tr.	tr.	2.5	0.45	3	0.54	22
Okra, cooked	8 pods	tr.	tr.	2	0.28	5	0.71	28
Onions, cooked	1/2c.	tr.	tr.	1	0.12	7	0.87	32
Parsley	1T.	tr.	tr.	tr.	tr.	tr.	tr.	tr.
Pepper, red, green	1 pepper	tr.	tr.	1	0.20	4	0.80	20
Radishes, small	4	tr.	tr.	tr.	tr.	1	1	4
Rutabagas	1/2c.	tr.	tr.	0.5	0.06	6.5	0.86	30
Sauerkraut, canned	1/2c.	tr.	tr.	1	0.16	5	0.83	24
Squash, summer	1/2c.	tr.	tr.	1	0.20	4	0.80	20
Tomato, medium	1	tr.	tr.	2	0.22	7	0.77	36
Tomato juice	1/2c.	tr.	tr.	1	0.16	5	0.83	24
Turnips, cooked	1/2c.	tr.	tr.	0.5	0.09	4	0.90	22
Vegetable juice	1/2c.	tr.	tr.	1	0.20	4	0.80	20
Watercress	1/2c.	tr.	tr.	1	0.33	2	0.66	12

PROTEIN FOODS

	PORTION	FAT		PROTEIN		CARB.		KCAL
		grams	%	grams	%	grams	%	
Beans, lima	1c.	1	0.05	12	0.26	32	0.71	180
Beans, red, canned	1c.	1	0.03	15	0.26	42	0.73	230
Beef:								
corned, canned	3 oz.	10	0.50	22	0.49	0	0	178
hamburger, lean	3 oz.	10	0.49	23	0.50	0	0	182
Roast, lean	2-1/2 oz.	3	0.21	24	0.78	0	0	123
round steak	1/2 oz.	4	0.30	21	0.70	0	0	120
sirloin steak	2 oz.	4	0.33	18	0.66	0	0	108
Cheese:								
blue	1 oz.	8	0.60	6	0.20	6	0.20	120
Cheddar	1 oz.	10	0.69	7	0.21	3	0.09	130
Colby	1 oz.	9	0.59	7	0.20	7	0.20	137
cottage, 2% fat	4 oz.	2	0.18	16	0.65	4	0.16	98
cream	1 oz.	10	0.90	2	0.16	0.7	0.02	100
Monterey	1 oz.	9	0.74	7	0.25	tr.	tr.	109
mozzarella	1 oz.	6	0.67	6	0.30	0.5	0.02	80
Parmesan	1 T.	2	0.78	2	0.34	tr.	tr.	23
ricotta, skim	1/2c.	10	0.52	14	0.32	6	0.14	170
processed American	1 oz.	9	0.76	6	0.22	tr.	tr.	106
processed Swiss	1 oz.	7	0.67	7	0.30	0.6	0.02	93
Egg	1 oz.	6	0.72	6	0.32	tr.	tr.	75
Fish:								
clams, canned	3 oz.	1	0.20	7	0.62	2	0.17	45
crab, canned	3 oz.	2	0.21	15	0.73	1	0.04	82
haddock	3 oz.	5	0.33	17	0.51	5	0.15	133
oysters, raw	8	2	0.24	10	0.54	4	0.21	74
perch	3 oz.	4	0.29	16	0.51	6	0.19	124
salmon, canned	3 oz.	5	0.39	17	0.60	0	0	113
sardines	1-1/2 oz.	4.50	0.50	10	0.50	0	0	80
shrimp	1-1/2 oz.	0.50	0.08	10	0.86	0.5	0.04	46
sole	3 oz.	0.60	0.06	14.1	0.93	0	0	60
tuna	1-1/2 oz.	3.50	0.40	12	0.60	0	0	79
Hot dogs	1	14	0.81	6	0.15	1	0.03	155
Lentils	1/2c.	0.50	0.02	10	0.27	26	0.70	148
Peanut butter	1 T.	8	0.74	4	0.14	3	0.11	109
Peas, split, cooked	1/2c.	0.50	0.02	10	0.27	26	0.70	148
Poultry, broil, skinned	3 oz.	3	0.25	20	0.74	0	0	107
Pork:								
chops, boned	2 oz.	7	0.51	15	0.48	0	0	123
ham, roast, lean	2 oz.	12	0.70	12	0.30	0	0	156
roast, lean	2-1/2 oz.	10	0.52	20	0.47	0	0	170
sausage	1 oz.	12	0.63	5	0.12	tr.	tr.	128

FRUITS

	PORTION	FAT		PROTEIN		CARB.		KCAL
		grams	%	grams	%	grams	%	
Apple, raw, medium	1	tr.	tr.	tr.	tr.	13	1	52
Apple juice	1c.	tr.	tr.	tr.	tr.	30	1	120
Applesauce, canned	1/2c.	tr.	tr.	0.5	0.01	30	0.99	120
Apricots, fresh	3	tr.	tr.	1	0.06	14	0.93	60
Apricots, dried	1/2c.	tr.	tr.	4	0.07	50	0.90	220
Banana, small	1	tr.	tr.	1	0.04	23	0.95	96
Blueberries	1/2c.	tr.	tr.	tr.	tr.	11	0.97	45
Cantaloupe	1/2c.	tr.	tr.	1	0.06	14	0.93	60
Cherries, sweet, raw	1/2c.	tr.	tr.	1	0.09	10	0.90	44
Dates	1/4c.	tr.	tr.	1	0.02	32.5	0.97	134
Figs, fresh, small	1	tr.	tr.	tr.	tr.	8	1	32
Figs, dried	1	tr.	tr.	1	0.06	15	0.93	64
Fruit cocktail	1/2c.	0.50	0.03	0.5	0.01	25	0.92	106
Grapefruit, fresh	1/2c.	tr.	tr.	0.5	0.04	11.5	0.95	48
Grapefruit juice	1/2c.	tr.	tr.	0.5	0.04	12	0.96	50
Grapes, American	12	0.50	0.10	0.5	0.05	8	0.86	37
Grape juice	1/2c.	tr.	tr.	0.5	0.02	21	0.97	86
Honeydew melon	1 wedge	tr.	tr.	1	0.07	12	0.92	52
Lemon juice, unsweet.	1T.	tr.	tr.	tr.	tr.	1.0	1	5
Mandarin oranges	1	1	0.20	1	0.08	8	0.71	45
Mango	1	tr.	tr.	1.6	0.03	39	0.96	162
Nectarine	1	tr.	tr.	1	0.04	24	0.96	100
Orange	1	tr.	tr.	1	0.05	16	0.94	68
Orange juice, fresh	1/2c.	tr.	tr.	1	0.07	13	0.92	56
Papaya	1/2	tr.	tr.			9	0.99	36
Peach, raw, medium	1	tr.	tr.	1	0.09	10	0.90	44
Pear, raw, medium	1	1	0.07	1	0.03	25	0.88	113
Persimmon, native	1	tr.	tr.	1	0.04	20	0.23	84
Pineapple, raw	1/2c.	tr.	tr.	0.5	0.04	10	0.95	42
Pineapple juice, canned	1/2c.	tr.	tr.	0.5	0.02	17	0.97	70
Plums	1	tr.	tr.	tr.	tr.	7	0.99	28
Prunes	2	tr.	tr.	0.5	0.05	9	0.94	38
Prune juice	0.50	tr.	tr.	0.5	0.02	25	0.98	102
Raisins	1 T.	tr.	tr.	0.5	0.03	15.5	0.96	64
Raspberries, unsweet.	1/2c.	0.50	0.09	0.5	0.04	9	0.85	42
Strawberries, unsweet.	1/2c.	0.50	0.11	0.5	0.05	7	0.82	34
Tangerine	1	tr.	tr.	1	0.09	10	0.90	44
Watermelon	1	tr.	tr.	0.5	0.04	10	0.95	42

INDEX